PROSTATE CANCER

Edited by **Cem Onal**

Prostate Cancer
http://dx.doi.org/10.5772/intechopen.70249
Edited by Cem Onal

Contributors

Bora Tas, Gazalla Ayub Shiekh, Hikmet Köseoğlu, Gunnel Hallden, Ahmed Ali, Alireza Ziaei

Notice

Statements and opinions expressed in the chapters are these of the individual contributors and not necessarily those of the editors or publisher. No responsibility is accepted for the accuracy of information contained in the published chapters. The publisher assumes no responsibility for any damage or injury to persons or property arising out of the use of any materials, instructions, methods or ideas contained in the book.

First published in London, United Kingdom, 2018 by IntechOpen
IntechOpen is the global imprint of INTECHOPEN LIMITED, registered in England and Wales, registration number: 11086078, The Shard, 25th floor, 32 London Bridge Street
London, SE19SG – United Kingdom
Printed in Croatia

British Library Cataloguing-in-Publication Data
A catalogue record for this book is available from the British Library

Additional hard copies can be obtained from orders@intechopen.com

Prostate Cancer, Edited by Cem Onal
p. cm.
Print ISBN 978-1-78923-999-7
Online ISBN 978-1-78984-000-1

We are IntechOpen,
the world's leading publisher of
Open Access books
Built by scientists, for scientists

3,700+
Open access books available

116,000+
International authors and editors

119M+
Downloads

151
Countries delivered to

Our authors are among the

Top 1%
most cited scientists

12.2%
Contributors from top 500 universities

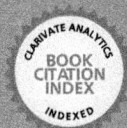

Interested in publishing with us?
Contact book.department@intechopen.com

Numbers displayed above are based on latest data collected.
For more information visit www.intechopen.com

Meet the editor

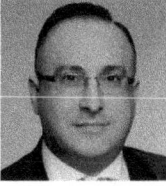

Dr. Onal is a founder physician of the Baskent University Adana Dr. Turgut Noyan Research and Treatment Center, Department of Radiation Oncology, Turkey, and is still serving as a professor and chair at the same institute. His main areas of interest are prostate cancer, breast cancer, and gynecological malignancies. He has great experience in prostate cancer treatments, especially IMRT and IGRT, gynecological tumor brachytherapy, stereotactic radiotherapy, and radiosurgery. Dr. Onal has approximately 100 international and national papers published in different journals, and approximately 200 international and national abstracts presented at different scientific meetings. He is peer-reviewing in 40 journals. Dr. Onal gives lectures on new radiotherapy facilities in different course programs conducted by the Turkish Society for Radiation Oncology.

Contents

Preface

It is my pleasure to present this book entitled *Prostate Cancer*. It brings together the experience of several researchers who dedicate many hours a day to treat prostate cancer patients.

This book comprises both diagnosis and treatment strategies of prostate cancer. Prostate cancer is the second most common cancer type and the fifth most common cause of cancer-related death in men. Although most patients are diagnosed with early stage and localized disease with excellent survival rates, less than 5% of prostate cancer patients had metastatic disease at diagnosis with a substantial 5-year survival rate of 25% to 30%. The mainstay of treatment is androgen deprivation therapy; however, several new agents that prolong survival and improve the quality of life have been approved for the treatment of metastatic castration-resistant prostate cancer, including abiraterone, enzalutamide, cabazitaxel, sipuleucel T, and radium-223. With new diagnostic tools and new treatment strategies, most prostate cancers are treated with conservative treatment strategies diagnosed at earlier stages.

The book is divided into two sections. The first section encompasses new diagnostic strategies and the second section encompasses new treatment strategies. This book is intended to bring forward the many advancements in prostate cancer diagnosis and treatment. There are many valuable contributions from physicians and medical physicists who are experts in their fields. I would like to thank all contributors for their kind efforts in the preparation of this book.

Cem Onal MD
Professor, Chair
Baskent University Faculty of Medicine
Adana Dr. Turgut Noyan Research and Treatment Center
Department of Radiation Oncology
Adana, Turkey

Diagnosis of Prostate Cancer

Chapter 1

Genetics in the Prostate Cancer

Hikmet Köseoğlu

Additional information is available at the end of the chapter

http://dx.doi.org/10.5772/intechopen.77259

Abstract

Any disruption in the intracellular functions ranging from DNA transcription to protein ligand binding as well as intercellular communication may cause cellular transformation to malignant cell in the proper microenvironment when it could escape from the immune system. In this chapter, specifically, genetic alterations playing role in the prostate cancer are intended to be reviewed briefly under the subheadings of genomic instability and the hallmarks of cancer which are sustaining proliferative signaling, evading growth suppressors, resisting cell death, enabling the replicative immortality, inducing angiogenesis, activating invasion and progression to metastatic disease, reprogramming of the energy metabolism and evading immune destruction.

Keywords: prostate, cancer, genetics, gene, carcinogenesis

1. Introduction

The basic molecular pathways and genetic alterations related to the cancer formation from normal cells irrespective of origin of tissue, are explained elsewhere in detail in many relevant textbooks. In this chapter, specifically, genetic alterations playing role in the prostate cancer are intended to be reviewed briefly under the subheadings of the hallmarks of cancer proposed by Hanahan and Weinberg, in the light of up to date studies [1, 2].

The proposed hallmarks of cancer are consisted of sustaining proliferative signaling, evading growth suppressors, resisting cell death, enabling replicative immortality, inducing angiogenesis, activating invasion and metastasis, reprogramming of energy metabolism and evading immune destruction [1, 2]. Underlying these hallmarks is the genome instability, which generates the genetic diversity promoting their acquisition [1, 2].

The Cancer Genome Atlas (TCGA) research on prostate cancer figured out seven genetic sub-types of prostate cancer [3]. Four subtypes are characterized by specific gene fusions includ-ing whereas the rest are characterized by genetic mutations particularly in SPOP, FOXA1, and IDH1 genes [3]. Gene fusions mainly included ERG (46%), ETV1 (8%), ETV4 (4%), FLI1 (1%) and gene mutations were commonly found in SPOP (11%), FOXA1 (3%) and IDH1 (1%) [3]. However, still almost quarter percent are not categorized in any of them, confirming genetic heterogenicity of prostate cancer [3]. However, these recently suggested genetic subgroups of prostate cancer may fit for future clinical trials of selective medical or genetic treatments in relevant subgroups. Yet, it is to be noted that the presented classification does not necessarily mean the relevant genes either involving gene fusions or mutations are themselves cause of cancer formation and yet they may only represent common alterations during carcinogenesis driven by any other one.

In other words; any disruption in the intracellular functions ranging from DNA transcrip-tion to protein ligand binding as well as intercellular communication may cause cellular transformation to malignant cell in the proper microenvironment when it could escape from immunity.

2. Genomic instability

Using allelotyping except the short arms of the acrocentric chromosomes, loss of heterozy-gosity and or gene fusions were shown to be 61% in prostate cancer [4]. Common allelic deletions were in chromosome 16q (60%), chromosome 8p (50%), chromosome 10p (55%) and 10q (30%). Allelic deletions of chromosomes 2, 3, 7, 12, 13, 17, 18, 22, X and Y were at lower frequencies, however no allelic deletions were present in any case without any of the dele-tions in chromosomes 8, 10, or 16 [4–7]. As expected, the more chromosomal deletions were present, the higher histological grade was present in prostate cancer [4]. This genetic het-erozygosity more has recently been confirmed by TCGA research as the gene fusions were reported in 59% of prostate cancer [3]. With more specific methods, deletion in some specific regions of chromosome 8p (specifically 8p11-8p21) is more common up to 50–70% in prostate cancer compared to others [4, 5, 8, 9]. Chromosomal region 8p11-8p21 contains over 400 genes (**Figure 1**) among which some has gained more attention in research for prostate carcinogen-esis like NKX3.1 which is an androgen regulated prostate specific homeobox gene [10–12]. Conditional deletion of one or both alleles of Nkx3.1 in mice has been shown to cause pros-tatic intraepithelial neoplasia (PIN) [13]. Even in murine epigenetic cancer models, Nkx3.1 deficiency further increased the frequency of PIN lesions [14].

Another chromosomal alteration commonly seen, occur in chromosome 10 [4, 5, 15–19]. One of the common alterations (60%) is the loss of the phosphatase and tensin homolog gene (PTEN) on chromosome 10q23.3 which is a negative regulator of the PIK3/Akt survival path-way [15–19]. The loss of PTEN in prostate cancer has been linked to higher Gleason grades, oncogenic TMPRSS2-ERG fusions, androgen-independent progression and metastasis [15–19]. Else, the size of PTEN deletions were classified into five distinct subtypes: (1) small interstitial (70 bp–789 kb); (2) large interstitial (1–7 MB); (3) large proximal (3–65 MB); (4) large terminal

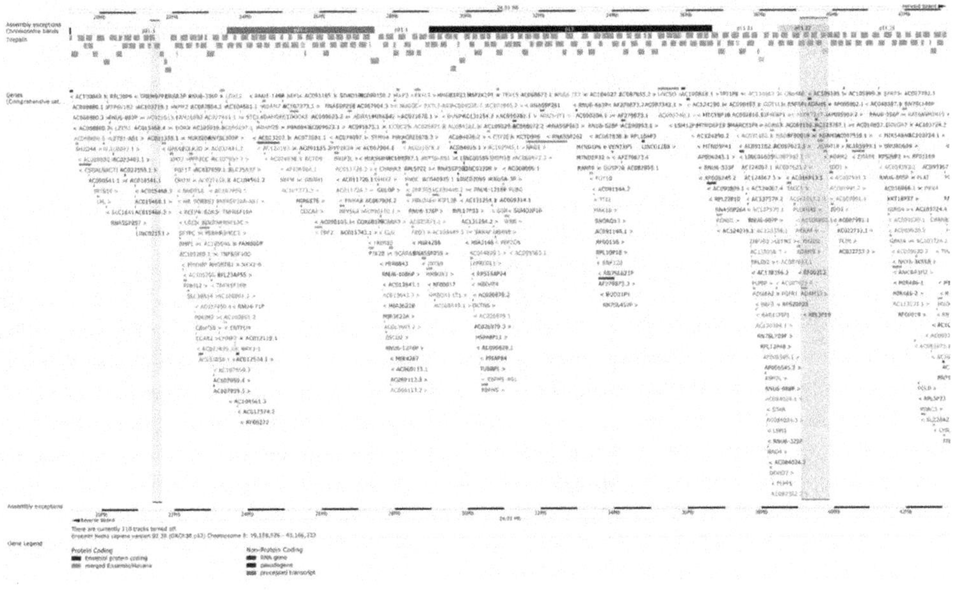

Figure 1. Some of the important genes located in 8p11-8p21 which are deleted up to 50–70% of prostate cancer (from http://www.ensembl.org).

(8–64 MB), and (5) extensive (71–132 MB), all were flanked by low copy repetitive (LCR) sequences [20]. All types had some gains of 3q21.1-3q29 and deletions at 8p, RB1, TP53 and TMPRSS2-ERG and ones with large interstitial deletion had worse prognosis [20]. Although PTEN deletions seem to affect aneuploidy through PIK3/Akt pathway, some other factors act directly. To give a sample, NKX3.1 binds to androgen receptor at the ERG gene breakpoint and inhibits the recombination of TMPRSS2 and ERG gene loci. Loss of NKX3.1 favors error-prone nonhomologous end-joining (NHEJ), further increasing TMPRSS2-ERG fusions [21]. Interestingly, intrinsic mechanism of the repair of DNA double-strand breaks (DSBs) driven by BRD4, itself may mediate the formation of oncogenic gene rearrangements by engaging the NHEJ pathway [22]. BRD4 belongs to the bromodomain and extra-terminal (BET) family of chromatin reader proteins that bind acetylated histones. These findings further outline importance of de novo alterations occurring synchronously are important for carcinogenesis together with error-prone intrinsic DNA repair mechanisms.

Again, the deletion of 16q23-q24 which is one of the most frequent genetic aberrations is associated with poor prognostic factors like advanced tumor stage, high Gleason grade, accelerated cell proliferation lymph node metastases and positive surgical margin [7, 23, 24]. Having ERG fusions were associated with higher incidence of 16q deletions [7, 23, 24]. Also, deletion of chromosome 13q occurs up to 50% of prostate cancer and its importance lies in the fact that this region contains RB transcriptional corepressor 1 gene which an important negative regulator of the cell cycle and the first tumor suppressor gene found [25, 26]. As well, deletion of three loci between 13q14.2 and 13q14.3 is associated with early biochemical relapse [27].

Other than structural chromosomal aberrations like aneuploidy, translocation, etc. epigenetics is another issue considered in carcinogenesis. The term "field cancerization" which had been suggested for head and neck cancers for the first time, refers to multifocal presence of genetic aberrations necessary for malignant transformation in a given tissue [28].

This term is also valid for prostate cancer, as cancerous tissues are multifocal with varying Gleason scores and preneoplastic tissues like high grade prostatic intraepithelial neoplasia (HGPIN) are detected closer to cancerous tissues [29]. This is further confirmed by methylation studies [30–35]. In a study comparing methylation status of GSTP1, MGMT, p14/ARF, p16/CDKN2A, RASSF1A, APC, TIMP3, S100A2 and CRBP1 genes among prostate cancer, HGPIN and BPH tissues, methylation was increased significantly from BPH to HGPIN and to prostate cancer [30]. Quantitative methylation specific PCR study of radical prostatectomy specimens, methylation of some genes like APC, RARb2 and RASSF1A were continuous in the histopathologically normal tissue around the cancerous tissue, forming a methylation halo up to 3 mm [31]. Another study including microarray study of methylation of large numbers of genes, the length of the halo was detected to be up to 10 mm [32].

3. Microenvironment

Prostatic stromal microenvironment is important for normal organogenesis as well as supporting carcinogenesis and the survival of the cancer cells [36, 37]. However, the exact pathways and stroma-tumoral interactions are poorly understood and still needed to be further clarified.

Cultured fibroblasts from regions close to prostate cancer cells were shown to induce tumor progression of initiated nontumorigenic epithelial cells both in an in vivo tissue recombination system and in an in vitro coculture system [38, 39]. Prostatic carcinoma-associated fibroblasts secrete SDF-1 which activates Akt pathway in the via the TGF-beta-regulated CXCR4 [40]. That is, TGF-beta promotes tumor formation although it has primarily growth-inhibitory action [40]. Marked reactive stroma is associated with poor prognosis in clinically localized prostate cancer and microarray gene expression analysis detected higher expression of 544 genes and lower expression of 606 genes in the reactive stroma, all of which have various functions like neurogenesis, axon genesis and DNA damage repair pathways [41]. In a recent study evaluating the nuclear and mitochondrial DNA integrity of prostate cancer cells, prostate cancer-associated stroma detected copy-neutral diploid genome with only rare and small somatic copy-number aberrations in contrast to several small somatic copy-number aberrations in prostate cancer cells [42]. This indicates, that above-mentioned gene expression changes in prostate cancer-adjacent stroma seem to be not related to frequent or recurrent genomic alterations in the tumor microenvironment [42].

Also, metabolic status of the prostatic stromal microenvironment has been suggested to influence the tumorigenic potential of the tumor epithelial compartment [43]. As well, it has been shown that the loss of the signaling adapter, p62, in stromal cells triggered an inflammatory response, activating cancer-associated fibroblasts which promotes tumor formation in vitro and in vivo. Loss of p62 resulted in lower mTORC1 activity and deregulation of metabolic pathways related to the inflammation [44].

One interesting study, chronic bacterial inflammation with inoculated *Escherichia coli* bacteria induced focal prostatic glandular atypia/ prostatic intraepithelial neoplasia in male C3H/HeOuJ mice, suggesting a link between inflammation and prostatic neoplasia [45].

4. Sustaining proliferative signaling

To keep normal tissue architecture and function normal cells need to control proliferative signaling. However, in cancer cells, proliferative signaling is sustained to keep their growth. This is accomplished by either increased paracrine stimulation or excessive response to hormones by altered receptor matching or deregulated pathways. Insulin has been shown to activate insulin activated the insulin receptor (INSR) in case of inhibition of the IGF1 receptor (IGF1R) [46]. Mitochondrial redox signaling by p66Shc-ROS pathway has been shown to promote androgen-induced prostate cancer cell proliferation. As well, dihydrotestosterone was shown to increase the translocation of p66Shc into mitochondria and its interaction with cytochrome c [47]. The phosphatidylinositol 3′-kinase (PI3K) pathway has been suggested to be a dominant growth factor-activated cell survival pathway in prostate carcinoma cells. Apoptosis induced by PI3K inhibition has been shown to be reduced by either dihydrotestosterone or ErbB1 activating ligands which are epidermal growth factor, transforming growth factor alpha, and heparin-binding EGF-like growth factor [48]. Smad1 acts as a substrate for MAPKs and plays a central role in transmitting signals from the pathways of bone morphogenetic proteins. Deregulation of the pathways of bone morphogenetic proteins and activation of the ERK/MAP kinase (MAPK) pathway by growth factors was suggested to promote the development and progression of prostate cancer [49].

5. Evading growth suppressors and resisting cell death

In general sense, cancer cells need to gain new capabilities to suppress or bypass cell cycle checkpoints that negatively regulate the cell proliferation and promote apoptosis. Chromosome 17p includes an important gene, TP53 which encodes a tumor suppressor protein, p53, containing transcriptional activation, DNA binding, and oligomerization domains and it functions in cellular stresses to induce cell cycle arrest, apoptosis, senescence, DNA repair, or changes in metabolism. Deletion of chromosome 17p occurs mainly in advanced stages of prostate cancer and metastatic prostate cancer rather that early invasive prostate cancer [50–52]. BCL2 gene located in 18q21.33, encodes an integral outer mitochondrial membrane protein which blocks apoptosis. Its overexpression occurs in advanced, hormone-refractory disease [53].

Functional loss of CDKN1B which maps to 12p13.1 is prevalent in prostate cancer [54]. It inhibits cyclin-dependent kinase (CDK), sharing similarity with another inhibitor CDKN1A/p21. The encoded protein prevents the activation of cyclin E-CDK2 or cyclin D-CDK4 complexes, in this way it controls the cell cycle progression at G1 stage. It is degraded through CDK dependent phosphorylation and subsequent ubiquitination by SCF complexes, permitting cellular transition from quiescence to the proliferative state. Its inactivation in prostate cancer is done by expression loss or increased degradation by abnormal phosphorylation and ubiquitinylating, rather than being mutated [55, 56].

Cyclin dependent kinase inhibitor 2A (CDKN2A) located in 9p21.3 encodes three alternatively spliced variants two of which encode structurally related isoforms functioning as inhibitors of CDK4 kinase and one variant functioning as stabilizer of the tumor suppressor protein p53. It is also rarely mutated in early prostate cancer, mainly mutated in advanced disease [57].

6. Enabling replicative immortality

Telomeres are located at the ends of eukaryotic linear chromosomes to protect chromosomes from end-to-end fusions and protect against the loss of terminal DNA during cell division [58]. Telomerase which is a ribonucleoprotein polymerase, maintains telomere length during cell divisions by addition of the telomere repeat TTAGGG [59]. Therefore, telomerase is also important for the maintenance of chromosomal stability and cellular immortality. The enzyme consists of a protein component with reverse transcriptase activity, telomerase reverse transcriptase (TERT) for adding telomeric DNA repeats onto chromosome ends and an RNA component (TERC) for adding telomeric DNA repeats onto chromosome ends [60, 61] Telomerase activity was detected in prostate cancer and high-grade prostatic intraepithelial neoplasia [62, 63]. Both TERT and TERC activities are important in telomere maintenance. Knockdown of TERC by siRNA has been shown to reduce proliferation of prostate cancer cells and increased TERC expression which is regulated by MYC, was detected in prostate cancer [64]. In benign prostatic hyperplasia, PIN and prostate cancer, high levels of telomere dysfunction were detected, and it was suggested that telomere dysfunction may play a role in carcinogenesis through genomic instability [65].

7. Inducing angiogenesis

As in any kind of tumoral tissue, tissue needs more blood supply as it grows uncontrolled. Therefore, cancer cells need to regulate pathways to induce angiogenesis. In prostate cancer related angiogenesis, ps20 which is a TGF-beta1-induced regulator of angiogenesis, has been suggested to promote endothelial cell migration and/or pericyte stabilization of newly formed vascular structures [66]. As well, stromal expression of connective tissue growth factor also promotes angiogenesis and therefore prostate cancer progression. Expression of CTGF in tumor-reactive stroma has been shown to induce increased micro-vessel density. CTGF which is also a downstream mediator of TGF-beta1 seem to be another important regulator of angiogenesis in the tumor-reactive stromal microenvironment [67].

8. Activating invasion and metastasis

Epithelial cancers progress to higher pathological grades of malignancy carcinomas and become locally invasive and metastatic to distant locations. This is termed as epithelial to mesenchymal cell transition during which the, the associated cancer cells alter their shape, their attachment to other cells and the extracellular matrix.

Abnormal increased expression of the mitochondrial ribosomal protein S18-2 has been shown to induce epithelial to mesenchymal cell transition in prostate cancer through the TWIST2/E-cadherin signaling and induce CXCR4-mediated migration of prostate cancer cells [68]. MiRNALet-7a has been shown to induce invasion of prostate cancer cells and induce migration by stimulating epithelial-mesenchymal transition through CCR7/MAPK pathway [69]. Interestingly, inactivation of the androgen receptor resulted in lower expression of a transcriptional repressor (SAM pointed domain-containing ETS transcription factor, SPDEF) of CCL2, which mediates epithelial to mesenchymal cell transition of the prostate cancer cells. That may explain progression to metastatic stage in a subset of castration resistant prostate cancer [70].

9. Reprogramming of energy metabolism

It has been shown that energy metabolism of early prostate cancers mainly depends on lipids and other energetic molecules for energy production and not on aerobic respiration or aerobic glycolysis (Warburg effect) [71]. Initially defined by Otto Warburg, the Warburg effect defines increased rate of glucose uptake, lactate production in proliferating cells in the presence of oxygen and fully functioning mitochondria [72]. The Warburg effect is the first defined energy metabolism of cancer cells energy [72]. However, in prostate cancer that is not the matter, as prostate cancer cells do not have increased glucose uptake except advanced stage disease [73].

In the advanced stages, reduced mtDNA content is a critical step in the metabolism restructuring for cancer cell progression. As, MtDNA depleted prostate cancer cells exhibit Warburg effect [74]. Reduced microRNA-132 (miR-132) expression was suggested to cause metabolic switch in prostate cancer cells by inhibiting Glut1 expression which results increased rate of lactate formation, cellular glucose uptake and the rapid growth of the cancer cells [75].

10. Evading immune destruction

The immune system acts a barrier to tumor formation and progression. The role of immune system is clear when increased malignancies in transplant patients is considered. In patients with renal transplants, genitourinary malignancies are the third most common malignancy after skin malignancies and lymphoproliferative disorders [76–78].

Cancer cell transfer extracellular vesicle-mediated estrogen receptor-binding fragment-associated antigen 9 (EBAG9) to their microenvironment promoting self-immune escape and further progression. EBAG9 suppresses T-cell infiltration into tumor in vivo and limits T-cell cytotoxicity [79]. Interestingly, the adaptive immune system was suggested to promote de novo prostate carcinogenesis in a human c-Myc transgenic mouse model [80]. Recently, tumoral exosome-immune cell cross-talk has been suggested [81]. Prostate-cancer-derived exosomal prostaglandin E2 (PGE2) was suggested to result impaired CD8+ T cell response immunosuppression via exosomal regulation of dendritic cell function [81]. Exosomal PGE2 triggered potently the expression of CD73, an ecto-5-nucleotidase responsible for AMP to adenosine hydrolysis, on dendritic cells. CD73 induction of dendritic cell resulted in an ATP-dependent inhibition of TNFα- and IL-12-production [81].

11. Conclusions

Above briefly mentioned properties of prostate cancer cells and related genes, genetic pathways and their interactions have still no specific clinical use in prostate cancer management.

Yet, we are too far to understand the exact genetic mechanisms underlying prostate carcinogenesis. But, it is sure that as we progress in further researches we will be more surprised to find out unknown interactions of supposed to be well known genetic mechanism.

Conflict of interest

There is conflict of interest.

Author details

Hikmet Köseoğlu[1,2]*

*Address all correspondence to: hikmet.koseoglu@gmail.com

1 Ministry of Health, Health Sciences University, Istanbul Education Research Hospital, Istanbul, Turkey

2 Istanbul University Aziz Sancar Institute of Experimental Medicine Department of Genetics, Istanbul, Turkey

References

[1] Hanahan D, Weinberg RA. The hallmarks of cancer. Cell. 2000;**100**(1):57-70

[2] Hanahan D, Weinberg RA. Hallmarks of cancer: The next generation. Cell. 2011;**144**(5): 646-674

[3] Cancer Genome Atlas Research N. The molecular taxonomy of primary prostate cancer. Cell. 2015;**163**(4):1011-1025

[4] Kunimi K, Bergerheim US, Larsson IL, Ekman P, Collins VP. Allelotyping of human prostatic adenocarcinoma. Genomics. 1991;**11**(3):530-536

[5] Bergerheim US, Kunimi K, Collins VP, Ekman P. Deletion mapping of chromosomes 8, 10, and 16 in human prostatic carcinoma. Genes, Chromosomes & Cancer. 1991;**3**(3):215-220

[6] Saramaki OR, Porkka KP, Vessella RL, Visakorpi T. Genetic aberrations in prostate cancer by microarray analysis. International Journal of Cancer. 2006;**119**(6):1322-1329

[7] Osman I, Scher H, Dalbagni G, Reuter V, Zhang ZF, Cordon-Cardo C. Chromosome 16 in primary prostate cancer: A microsatellite analysis. International Journal of Cancer. 1997;**71**(4):580-584

[8] Chang M, Tsuchiya K, Batchelor RH, Rabinovitch PS, Kulander BG, Haggitt RC, et al. Deletion mapping of chromosome 8p in colorectal carcinoma and dysplasia arising in ulcerative colitis, prostatic carcinoma, and malignant fibrous histiocytomas. The American Journal of Pathology. 1994;**144**(1):1-6

[9] Matsuyama H, Pan Y, Skoog L, Tribukait B, Naito K, Ekman P, et al. Deletion mapping of chromosome 8p in prostate cancer by fluorescence in situ hybridization. Oncogene. 1994;**9**(10):3071-3076

[10] Bowen C, Bubendorf L, Voeller HJ, Slack R, Willi N, Sauter G, et al. Loss of NKX3.1 expression in human prostate cancers correlates with tumor progression. Cancer Research. 2000;**60**(21):6111-6115

[11] He WW, Sciavolino PJ, Wing J, Augustus M, Hudson P, Meissner PS, et al. A novel human prostate-specific, androgen-regulated homeobox gene (NKX3.1) that maps to 8p21, a region frequently deleted in prostate cancer. Genomics. 1997;**43**(1):69-77

[12] Ornstein DK, Cinquanta M, Weiler S, Duray PH, Emmert-Buck MR, Vocke CD, et al. Expression studies and mutational analysis of the androgen regulated homeobox gene NKX3.1 in benign and malignant prostate epithelium. The Journal of Urology. 2001;**165**(4):1329-1334

[13] Abdulkadir SA, Magee JA, Peters TJ, Kaleem Z, Naughton CK, Humphrey PA, et al. Conditional loss of Nkx3.1 in adult mice induces prostatic intraepithelial neoplasia. Molecular and Cellular Biology. 2002;**22**(5):1495-1503

[14] Damaschke NA, Yang B, Bhusari S, Avilla M, Zhong W, Blute ML Jr, et al. Loss of Igf2 gene imprinting in murine prostate promotes widespread neoplastic growth. Cancer Research. 2017;**77**(19):5236-5247

[15] Yoshimoto M, Ding K, Sweet JM, Ludkovski O, Trottier G, Song KS, et al. PTEN losses exhibit heterogeneity in multifocal prostatic adenocarcinoma and are associated with higher Gleason grade. Modern Pathology. 2013;**26**(3):435-447

[16] Phin S, Moore MW, Cotter PD. Genomic rearrangements of PTEN in prostate cancer. Frontiers in Oncology. 2013;**3**:240

[17] Murphy SJ, Karnes RJ, Kosari F, Castellar BE, Kipp BR, Johnson SH, et al. Integrated analysis of the genomic instability of PTEN in clinically insignificant and significant prostate cancer. Modern Pathology. 2016;29(2):143-156

[18] Gao T, Mei Y, Sun H, Nie Z, Liu X, Wang S. The association of phosphatase and tensin homolog (PTEN) deletion and prostate cancer risk: A meta-analysis. Biomedicine & Pharmacotherapy. 2016;83:114-121

[19] Bismar TA, Yoshimoto M, Vollmer RT, Duan Q, Firszt M, Corcos J, et al. PTEN genomic deletion is an early event associated with ERG gene rearrangements in prostate cancer. BJU International. 2011;107(3):477-485

[20] Vidotto T, Tiezzi DG, Squire JA. Distinct subtypes of genomic PTEN deletion size influence the landscape of aneuploidy and outcome in prostate cancer. Molecular Cytogenetics. 2018;11:1

[21] Bowen C, Zheng T, Gelmann EP. NKX3.1 suppresses TMPRSS2-ERG gene rearrangement and mediates repair of androgen receptor-induced DNA damage. Cancer Research. 2015;75(13):2686-2698

[22] Li X, Baek G, Ramanand SG, Sharp A, Gao Y, Yuan W, et al. BRD4 promotes DNA repair and mediates the formation of TMPRSS2-ERG gene rearrangements in prostate cancer. Cell Reports. 2018;22(3):796-808

[23] Kluth M, Runte F, Barow P, Omari J, Abdelaziz ZM, Paustian L, et al. Concurrent deletion of 16q23 and PTEN is an independent prognostic feature in prostate cancer. International Journal of Cancer. 2015;137(10):2354-2363

[24] Harkonen P, Kyllonen AP, Nordling S, Vihko P. Loss of heterozygosity in chromosomal region 16q24.3 associated with progression of prostate cancer. The Prostate. 2005;62(3):267-274

[25] Cooney KA, Wetzel JC, Merajver SD, Macoska JA, Singleton TP, Wojno KJ. Distinct regions of allelic loss on 13q in prostate cancer. Cancer Research. 1996;56(5):1142-1145

[26] Li C, Larsson C, Futreal A, Lancaster J, Phelan C, Aspenblad U, et al. Identification of two distinct deleted regions on chromosome 13 in prostate cancer. Oncogene. 1998;16(4):481-487

[27] Brookman-Amissah N, Nariculam J, Freeman A, Willamson M, Kirby RS, Masters JR, et al. Allelic imbalance at 13q14.2 approximately q14.3 in localized prostate cancer is associated with early biochemical relapse. Cancer Genetics and Cytogenetics. 2007;179(2):118-126

[28] Slaughter DP, Southwick HW, Smejkal W. Field cancerization in oral stratified squamous epithelium; clinical implications of multicentric origin. Cancer. 1953;6(5):963-968

[29] Qian J, Wollan P, Bostwick DG. The extent and multicentricity of high-grade prostatic intraepithelial neoplasia in clinically localized prostatic adenocarcinoma. Human Pathology. 1997;28(2):143-148

[30] Jeronimo C, Henrique R, Hoque MO, Mambo E, Ribeiro FR, Varzim G, et al. A quantitative promoter methylation profile of prostate cancer. Clinical Cancer Research. 2004;**10**(24):8472-8478

[31] Mehrotra J, Varde S, Wang H, Chiu H, Vargo J, Gray K, et al. Quantitative, spatial resolution of the epigenetic field effect in prostate cancer. The Prostate. 2008;**68**(2):152-160

[32] Yang B, Bhusari S, Kueck J, Weeratunga P, Wagner J, Leverson G, et al. Methylation profiling defines an extensive field defect in histologically normal prostate tissues associated with prostate cancer. Neoplasia. 2013;**15**(4):399-408

[33] Van Neste L, Bigley J, Toll A, Otto G, Clark J, Delree P, et al. A tissue biopsy-based epigenetic multiplex PCR assay for prostate cancer detection. BMC Urology. 2012;**12**:16

[34] Wojno KJ, Costa FJ, Cornell RJ, Small JD, Pasin E, Van Criekinge W, et al. Reduced rate of repeated prostate biopsies observed in ConfirmMDx clinical utility field study. American Health & Drug Benefits. 2014;**7**(3):129-134

[35] Stewart GD, Van Neste L, Delvenne P, Delree P, Delga A, McNeill SA, et al. Clinical utility of an epigenetic assay to detect occult prostate cancer in histopathologically negative biopsies: Results of the MATLOC study. The Journal of Urology. 2013;**189**(3):1110-1116

[36] Li H, Fan X, Houghton J. Tumor microenvironment: The role of the tumor stroma in cancer. Journal of Cellular Biochemistry. 2007;**101**(4):805-815

[37] Taylor RA, Risbridger GP. Prostatic tumor stroma: A key player in cancer progression. Current Cancer Drug Targets. 2008;**8**(6):490-497

[38] Olumi AF, Dazin P, Tlsty TD. A novel coculture technique demonstrates that normal human prostatic fibroblasts contribute to tumor formation of LNCaP cells by retarding cell death. Cancer Research. 1998;**58**(20):4525-4530

[39] Olumi AF, Grossfeld GD, Hayward SW, Carroll PR, Tlsty TD, Cunha GR. Carcinoma-associated fibroblasts direct tumor progression of initiated human prostatic epithelium. Cancer Research. 1999;**59**(19):5002-5011

[40] Ao M, Franco OE, Park D, Raman D, Williams K, Hayward SW. Cross-talk between paracrine-acting cytokine and chemokine pathways promotes malignancy in benign human prostatic epithelium. Cancer Research. 2007;**67**(9):4244-4253

[41] Dakhova O, Ozen M, Creighton CJ, Li R, Ayala G, Rowley D, et al. Global gene expression analysis of reactive stroma in prostate cancer. Clinical Cancer Research. 2009;**15**(12):3979-3989

[42] Bianchi-Frias D, Basom R, Delrow JJ, Coleman IM, Dakhova O, Qu X, et al. Cells comprising the prostate cancer microenvironment lack recurrent clonal somatic genomic aberrations. Molecular Cancer Research. 2016;**14**(4):374-384

[43] Lisanti MP, Martinez-Outschoorn UE, Sotgia F. Oncogenes induce the cancer-associated fibroblast phenotype: Metabolic symbiosis and "fibroblast addiction" are new therapeutic targets for drug discovery. Cell Cycle. 2013;**12**(17):2723-2732

[44] Valencia T, Kim JY, Abu-Baker S, Moscat-Pardos J, Ahn CS, Reina-Campos M, et al. Metabolic reprogramming of stromal fibroblasts through p62-mTORC1 signaling promotes inflammation and tumorigenesis. Cancer Cell. 2014;**26**(1):121-135

[45] Elkahwaji JE, Hauke RJ, Brawner CM. Chronic bacterial inflammation induces prostatic intraepithelial neoplasia in mouse prostate. British Journal of Cancer. 2009;**101**(10): 1740-1748

[46] Weinstein D, Sarfstein R, Laron Z, Werner H. Insulin receptor compensates for IGF1R inhibition and directly induces mitogenic activity in prostate cancer cells. Endocr Connect. 2014;**3**(1):24-35

[47] Veeramani S, Yuan TC, Lin FF, Lin MF. Mitochondrial redox signaling by p66Shc is involved in regulating androgenic growth stimulation of human prostate cancer cells. Oncogene. 2008;**27**(37):5057-5068

[48] Lin J, Adam RM, Santiestevan E, Freeman MR. The phosphatidylinositol 3'-kinase pathway is a dominant growth factor-activated cell survival pathway in LNCaP human prostate carcinoma cells. Cancer Research. 1999;**59**(12):2891-2897

[49] Qiu T, Grizzle WE, Oelschlager DK, Shen X, Cao X. Control of prostate cell growth: BMP antagonizes androgen mitogenic activity with incorporation of MAPK signals in Smad1. The EMBO Journal. 2007;**26**(2):346-357

[50] Saric T, Brkanac Z, Troyer DA, Padalecki SS, Sarosdy M, Williams K, et al. Genetic pattern of prostate cancer progression. International Journal of Cancer. 1999;**81**(2):219-224

[51] Brooks JD, Bova GS, Ewing CM, Piantadosi S, Carter BS, Robinson JC, et al. An uncertain role for p53 gene alterations in human prostate cancers. Cancer Research. 1996;**56**(16):3814-3822

[52] Voeller HJ, Sugars LY, Pretlow T, Gelmann EP. p53 oncogene mutations in human prostate cancer specimens. The Journal of Urology. 1994;**151**(2):492-495

[53] McDonnell TJ, Navone NM, Troncoso P, Pisters LL, Conti C, von Eschenbach AC, et al. Expression of bcl-2 oncoprotein and p53 protein accumulation in bone marrow metastases of androgen independent prostate cancer. The Journal of Urology. 1997;**157**(2):569-574

[54] Macri E, Loda M. Role of p27 in prostate carcinogenesis. Cancer Metastasis Reviews. 1998;**17**(4):337-344

[55] Cordon-Cardo C, Koff A, Drobnjak M, Capodieci P, Osman I, Millard SS, et al. Distinct altered patterns of p27KIP1 gene expression in benign prostatic hyperplasia and prostatic carcinoma. Journal of the National Cancer Institute. 1998;**90**(17):1284-1291

[56] Iacopino F, Angelucci C, Lama G, Zelano G, La Torre G, D'Addessi A, et al. Apoptosis-related gene expression in benign prostatic hyperplasia and prostate carcinoma. Anticancer Research. 2006;**26**(3A):1849-1854

[57] Gu K, Mes-Masson AM, Gauthier J, Saad F. Analysis of the p16 tumor suppressor gene in early-stage prostate cancer. Molecular Carcinogenesis. 1998;**21**(3):164-170

[58] Blackburn EH. Telomeres and telomerase: The means to the end (Nobel lecture). Angewandte Chemie (International Ed. in English). 2010;**49**(41):7405-7421

[59] Greider CW, Blackburn EH. Identification of a specific telomere terminal transferase activity in Tetrahymena extracts. Cell. 1985;**43**(2 Pt 1):405-413

[60] Feng J, Funk WD, Wang SS, Weinrich SL, Avilion AA, Chiu CP, et al. The RNA component of human telomerase. Science. 1995;**269**(5228):1236-1241

[61] Greider CW, Blackburn EH. A telomeric sequence in the RNA of Tetrahymena telomerase required for telomere repeat synthesis. Nature. 1989;**337**(6205):331-337

[62] Lin Y, Uemura H, Fujinami K, Hosaka M, Harada M, Kubota Y. Telomerase activity in primary prostate cancer. The Journal of Urology. 1997;**157**(3):1161-1165

[63] Zhang W, Kapusta LR, Slingerland JM, Klotz LH. Telomerase activity in prostate cancer, prostatic intraepithelial neoplasia, and benign prostatic epithelium. Cancer Research. 1998;**58**(4):619-621

[64] Baena-Del Valle JA, Zheng Q, Esopi DM, Rubenstein M, Hubbard GK, Moncaliano MC, et al. MYC drives overexpression of telomerase RNA (hTR/TERC) in prostate cancer. The Journal of Pathology. 2018;**244**(1):11-24

[65] Tu L, Huda N, Grimes BR, Slee RB, Bates AM, Cheng L, et al. Widespread telomere instability in prostatic lesions. Molecular Carcinogenesis. 2016;**55**(5):842-852

[66] McAlhany SJ, Ressler SJ, Larsen M, Tuxhorn JA, Yang F, Dang TD, et al. Promotion of angiogenesis by ps20 in the differential reactive stroma prostate cancer xenograft model. Cancer Research. 2003;**63**(18):5859-5865

[67] Yang F, Tuxhorn JA, Ressler SJ, McAlhany SJ, Dang TD, Rowley DR. Stromal expression of connective tissue growth factor promotes angiogenesis and prostate cancer tumorigenesis. Cancer Research. 2005;**65**(19):8887-8895

[68] Mushtaq M, Jensen L, Davidsson S, Grygoruk OV, Andren O, Kashuba V, et al. The MRPS18-2 protein levels correlate with prostate tumor progression and it induces CXCR4-dependent migration of cancer cells. Scientific Reports. 2018;**8**(1):2268

[69] Tang G, Du R, Tang Z, Kuang Y. MiRNALet-7a mediates prostate cancer PC-3 cell invasion, migration by inducing epithelial-mesenchymal transition through CCR7/MAPK pathway. Journal of Cellular Biochemistry. 2018;**119**(4):3725-3731

[70] Tsai YC, Chen WY, Abou-Kheir W, Zeng T, Yin JJ, Bahmad H, et al. Androgen deprivation therapy-induced epithelial-mesenchymal transition of prostate cancer through downregulating SPDEF and activating CCL2. Biochimica et Biophysica Acta. 2018;**1864**:1717-1727

[71] Sadeghi RN, Karami-Tehrani F, Salami S. Targeting prostate cancer cell metabolism: Impact of hexokinase and CPT-1 enzymes. Tumour Biology. 2015;**36**(4):2893-2905

[72] Warburg O, Wind F, Negelein E. The metabolism of tumors in the body. The Journal of General Physiology. 1927;**8**(6):519-530

[73] Dueregger A, Schopf B, Eder T, Hofer J, Gnaiger E, Aufinger A, et al. Differential utilization of dietary fatty acids in benign and malignant cells of the prostate. PLoS One. 2015;**10**(8):e0135704

[74] Li X, Zhong Y, Lu J, Axcrona K, Eide L, Syljuasen RG, et al. MtDNA depleted PC3 cells exhibit Warburg effect and cancer stem cell features. Oncotarget. 2016;**7**(26):40297-40313

[75] Qu W, Ding SM, Cao G, Wang SJ, Zheng XH, Li GH. miR-132 mediates a metabolic shift in prostate cancer cells by targeting Glut1. FEBS Open Bio. 2016;**6**(7):735-741

[76] Penn I. The changing pattern of posttransplant malignancies. Transplantation Proceedings. 1991;**23**(1 Pt 2):1101-1103

[77] Penn I. Posttransplant malignancies. Transplantation Proceedings. 1999;**31**(1-2):1260-1262

[78] Villeneuve PJ, Schaubel DE, Fenton SS, Shepherd FA, Jiang Y, Mao Y. Cancer incidence among Canadian kidney transplant recipients. American Journal of Transplantation. 2007;**7**(4):941-948

[79] Miyazaki T, Ikeda K, Sato W, Horie-Inoue K, Inoue S. Extracellular vesicle-mediated EBAG9 transfer from cancer cells to tumor microenvironment promotes immune escape and tumor progression. Oncogene. 2018;**7**(1):7

[80] Melis MHM, Nevedomskaya E, van Burgsteden J, Cioni B, van Zeeburg HJT, Song JY, et al. The adaptive immune system promotes initiation of prostate carcinogenesis in a human c-Myc transgenic mouse model. Oncotarget. 2017;**8**(55):93867-93877

[81] Salimu J, Webber J, Gurney M, Al-Taei S, Clayton A, Tabi Z. Dominant immunosuppression of dendritic cell function by prostate-cancer-derived exosomes. Journal of Extracellular Vesicles. 2017;**6**(1):1368823

Advances in Medical Imaging Technology for Accurate Detection of Prostate Cancer

Alireza Ziaei

Additional information is available at the end of the chapter

http://dx.doi.org/10.5772/intechopen.77327

Abstract

Prostate cancer (PCa) is the most frequently diagnosed non-cutaneous male malignancy and one of the leading causes of cancer-related mortality in the United States. Biologic heterogeneity of PCa results is different presentations ranging from indolent to highly aggressive tumors with high morbidity and mortality. Due to this broad range of clinical behavior, it is required to differentiate clinically significant PCa (csPCa) tumors and reduce detection of indolent cancers. PCa is generally diagnosed with non-targeted systematic trans-rectal ultrasound (TRUS)-guided biopsy in patients with elevated prostate serum antigen (PSA) or abnormal digital rectal examination (DRE). Non-targeted systematic TRUS as the typical imaging modality for assessing the prostate, samples only a small part of the gland with a high possibly that the biopsy results may not catch the most aggressive tumor in the gland accurately. Multi-parametric (MP) magnetic resonance imaging (MRI), as the most specific and sensitive imaging modality in PCa management, has been reported to be the reference standard for prostate imaging endorsed. However, there are a variety of interpretive pitfalls, which have been reported to be encountered at mpMRI of the prostate. The purpose of this chapter is to provide a summary of the current advances in accurate detection of PCa.

Keywords: prostate cancer (PCa), prostate specific antigen, digital rectal exam, trans-rectal ultrasound guided biopsy (TRUSgBX), Gleason scores, multi-parametric (MP) magnetic resonance imaging (MRI)

1. Introduction

Prostate cancer (PCa) is the most frequently diagnosed non-cutaneous male malignancy and one of the leading causes of cancer-related mortality in the United States [1–3]. PCa is a disease of increasing significance in the world. Even though PCa may be less common in many developing countries, but its incidence and mortality rate has been raised [4]. The incidence of PCa influenced by the diagnostic efforts and the mortalities reported for any specific geographic region depending on the reliability of cancer detected [5]. The range of the five-year survival rate varies from 29% in patients with metastatic PCa to 100% in patients with localized disease [6, 7]. Biologic heterogeneity of PCa results is different presentations ranging from indolent to highly aggressive tumors with high morbidity and mortality [8] that affects the therapy, response, and prognosis of patients with PCa. Due to this broad range of clinical behavior, it is required to differentiate clinically significant prostate cancers (csPCa) tumors, defined as presence of Gleason pattern >4 and/or tumor volume > 0.5 ccs, and reduce detection of indolent cancers [9], since candidates for therapy from clinically insignificant tumors that can undergo active surveillance without any harm. Traditional treatment of PCa varies from radical prostatectomy (RP) or radiotherapy (RT) to watchful waiting [10, 11]. When prostate specific antigen (PSA) tests became beneficial for PCa screening, the United States gained a huge increase in the incidence of the disease [12]. Several years ago, many PCa were detected during the pathological exam of specimens from trans-urethral prostatectomies. These patients underwent surgery for benign prostatic hyperplasia (BPH), but up to 25% were found to have malignancy [13, 14]. However, the frequency of detecting such incidental cancers has gone down since PSA came into existence, as most of the men undergoing surgery for BPH have their PSA tested.

PCa is generally diagnosed with non-targeted systematic trans-rectal ultrasound (TRUS)-guided biopsy in patients with elevated PSA or abnormal digital rectal examination (DRE).

2. Prostate cancer diagnosis

2.1. Prostate specific antigen (PSA)

PSA is a natural enzyme that is produced entirely by the prostatic epithelial cells and is used as a marker for PCa. However, PSA is not cancer-specific as BPH, prostatitis and other urinary symptoms may elevate PSA levels. There is no absolute PSA level which indicates PCa and there is no PSA level below, which a man is assured not to have PCa, although higher PSA is associated with risk of PCa [15]. Traditionally, a level ≥ 4 ng/ml has been well-known as suspicious of PCa that indicated the need for biopsies. However, at this level, only about 30% of men with elevated levels will have PCA and normal levels may falsely exclude the presence of PCa, suggesting that PSA should not be used to exclude or diagnose PCa [16–20].

2.2. Digital rectal exam (DRE)

DRE is an essential part of the clinical exam of the patient when a tumor is palpable. Over 70% of lesions are located in the peripheral zone (PZ) and are palpable when they are bigger than a certain size [21]. Twenty-five percent of the tumors are located in the transitional zone (TZ) and cannot be reachable by DRE because of their location. Other than that as PCa is now detected at smaller tumor volumes and earlier stages, the number of palpable tumors is significantly reduced. This decreases sensitivity and specificity of the DRE [22–25]. Suspicious outcomes at DRE are an indicator of more aggressive PCa [26, 27] and trigger the need for prostate biopsies [27].

2.3. TRUS and TRUS guided biopsy (TRUSgBX)

TRUS is the typical imaging modality for assessing the prostate. Histological examination of 10–12 TRUSgBX cores from standard zones in the prostate is a gold standard for diagnosis of PCa [28]. Prostate biopsies have played a role from pure cancer detection to clinical management in the past several years. TRUS is typically the best way for measuring the volume of the prostate gland as well as guiding the biopsy needle; however, it lacks in both specificity and sensitivity for detection of PCa [28, 29]. Most of the lesions appear hypoechoic compared to the normal PZ; but some lesions are barely visible since about half of the cancer lesions are iso-echoic [29, 30] and cannot be detected. In addition, evaluation of the TZ on TRUS is limited because of the heterogeneity in the appearance caused by BPH making it difficult to detect especially the tumors located anteriorly. Thus, there is a considerable risk that a tumor is either being missed or the aggressive part of the tumor is not picked by the systematic biopsies. This may result in either repeated biopsies or incorrect Gleason score (GS).

TRUS guided prostate biopsy samples only a small part of the gland with a high possibility that the biopsy results may not catch the most aggressive tumor in the gland accurately [31, 32]. Non-targeted TRUSgBX usually takes 6–12 core biopsies of the PZ, which harbors about 70% of PCa [33]. The limitations of non-targeted TRUSgBX are well discussed in the recent year studies [34] with over 20% of false negative rate [35–37]. Also, non-targeted TRUSgBX may not provide accurate information about the volume and aggressiveness of PCa. It's been reported in some recent studies that after RP, 30–45% of the patients are upstaged from their initial diagnosis at TRUSgBX [38]. The anterior gland, TZ, and apex of the gland, which are recognized as areas with high possibilities of containing csPCa, are known to be under/not-sampled at standard TRUSgBX [39]. Since treatment protocol is completely based on risk stratification and depend on accurate GS, these limitations are very critical. It also leads to over-diagnosis of indolent PCa, which provides no benefit to the patients, and under-diagnoses of clinically significant tumors, which potentially harms patients. It has been reported that approximately 60% of patients with a diagnosis of indolent tumor choose aggressive treatment options such as RP, leading to numerous complications [40, 41]. The biopsies can also result in complications including bleeding and infections [42, 43]. Endoscopic ultrasound-guided fine needle aspiration (EUS-FNA) biopsy requires sedation and is associated with significant risks of complications such as pancreatitis, bowel perforation, and aspiration, which can be fatal [44]. In addition, confounding issue with needle biopsy is that most of the tumor mass is made up of stromal cells, not the epithelial cancer cells. Despite being the gold standard, EUS-FNA only has a sensitivity of 75–94% and a specificity of 78–95% [45]. The current diagnostic paradigm for PCa diagnosis has low diagnostic accuracy when they are associated with significant risk and cost [46].

3. Gleason scores (GS) for grading PCa

The histopathological aggressiveness of PCa is graded by the GS [47, 48]. The cancer tissue is graded on a scale from 1 to 5 based on the appearance of the cancerous cells and histo-pathological arrangement. This discrepancy between cancer and normal tissue reflects the aggressiveness of cancer. Since more than one class of Gleason grade is usually present in the biopsy tissue, a combination GS (ranging from 2 to 10) combining the dominant and the highest grade is assigned. The GS is intensely correlated to the clinical characteristics of the tumor and is a potent prognostic factor for treatment response. High GS indicates increased tumor aggressiveness and increased risk of tumor spread with a worse prognosis [49–52]. Hence, it has been suggested to divide the GS into risk groups based on the risk of metastasis and progression [53]. The risk assessment of a patient with diagnosed PCa and the treatment plan is highly based on the GS from TRUSgBX, which can be inaccurate because of sampling error, considering that the GS is upgraded in about 30% of the patient after RP [54]. Incorrect biopsy reported GS can result in incorrect risk stratification and possible under or over-treatment. The change of the reported GS during the past years with broadening of the Gleason grade 4 criteria [55] to improve the correlation between biopsy and RP GSs has resulted in a significant upgrade of tumor GS and made it difficult to compare pathological data over time. GS, as one of the best indicators of PCa, is a strong determinant of treatment selection. RP GS is an established prognostic indicator for recurrence of the disease. Therefore, accurate prediction of the final RP GS is critical. Clinical staging of PCa is based on the TNM classification [55, 56].

4. Magnetic resonance imaging (MRI) of the prostate

MRI of the prostate is performed on 1.5–3.0 Tesla MRI scanners combined with a pelvic phased-array coil placed over the pelvis with or without an endorectal coil (ERC) depending on the clinical situation. ERC, which is placed in the rectum just posterior to the prostate gland, reduces motion artifacts, and enhances image quality; but it has some disadvantages including increased scan time, increased costs, and reduced patient compliance because of the location of the coil in the rectum. The majority of prostatic MRI examinations can be performed with acceptable image quality without an ERC because of the increased spatial resolution (the ability to separate two dense structures from each other) and the increased signal-to-noise ratio on 3.0 T MRI. However, several studies reported improved image quality and diagnostic performance with an ERC [57, 58]. The European society of urogenital radiology's (ESUR) MR prostate guidelines states that the use of an ERC is optional for detection and preferable for staging at 3.0 T MRI [59].

4.1. Multi-parametric MRI (mpMRI)

Multi-parametric (MP) MRI, as the most specific and sensitive imaging modality in PCa management, has been reported to be the reference standard for prostate imaging endorsed [60, 61]. While TRUSgBX evaluates a limited piece of the prostate gland, magnetic resonance (MR) images provide detailed information about the whole prostate gland and potentially may be more accurate than random TRUSgBX [62]. The development of mp-MRI provides new possibilities in detection, characterization of the lesson and staging of PCa due to its high resolution and soft-tissue contrast [62]. Recently published data [62–67] indicates the rapidly growing use of mpMRI as the most specific and sensitive diagnostic imaging modality for PCa management. MpMRI provides detailed information about the morphological, metabolic, and cellular changes in the prostate as well as characterize tissue vascularity and correlate it to tumor aggressiveness [68, 69]. MP MRI sequences include high-resolution anatomical T2-weighted (T2W) and T1-weighted (T1W) images in combination with one or more functional MRI techniques such as diffusion-weighted imaging (DWI) and dynamic contrast-enhanced (DCE) imaging [63]. Two recently reported meta-analyses revealed that mpMRI has a high negative predictive value (NPV) for the detection of csPCa [70, 71], and it has been shown that mpMRI can estimate grade of PCa compared to histopathology results with a high degree of accuracy [72, 73]. Being noninvasive, a pathway with mpMRI as a predicting test in order to determine, which men with an elevated PSA undergo biopsy might reduce unnecessary biopsies, which are the pitfalls of routine screening practice and improve detection and diagnostic accuracy.

4.2. Multi-parametric MRI (mpMRI) pitfalls

There are several interpretive pitfalls, which have been reported [74] to be encountered at mpMRI of the prostate: Normal anatomic structures can mimic anterior and TZ located lesions; post-biopsy hemorrhage can mimic PZ PCa on T2W MRI; BPH resembles TZ PCa; acute and chronic prostatitis mimics PCa; ductal variant adenocarcinoma may be occult on T2W MRI. Moreover, technical pitfalls may be encountered at MP-MRI of the prostate: T2W motion correction with radial acquisition obscures some PCa; visual/quantitative analysis of DWI for tumor detection/grading is complex; DCE lacks standardization and is limited in the TZ; targeted biopsy of MR-detected lesions using TRUS-guidance is challenging. A failure to recognize and correct these types of errors may result in suboptimal care. False positive diagnoses of areas of potential cancers at mpMRI generate clinical uncertainty and often lead to multiple pointless biopsies or in certain cases surgical management of low-grade disease. Failure to recognize clinically significant cancers in males could result in suboptimal patient outcomes [74].

4.3. Accuracy of mpMRI

A study by Borofsky et al. [75] showed that of the 162 lesions, 136 (84%) were correctly identified with mpMRI and 16% were missed. In their study, among the lesions missed at mpMRI, GS was 3 + 4 in 17 (65%), 4 + 3 in one (4%), 4 + 4 in seven (27%), and 4 + 5 in one (4%). They reported that mpMRI has excellent sensitivity in the detection of PCa on an overall patient basis; however, a substantial number of cancers are missed either because lesions are not apparent or because they are too subtle for detection. Of those missed lesions, 58% were not visualized or were characterized as benign findings even at the second-look evaluation. They conclude that clinically important lesions can be missed, or their size can be underestimated at mpMRI [75]. Some previous studies also showed that in some cases tumors were invisible including lesions with pathologic GS greater than 3 + 4 and pathologic volume of more than 0.5 mL [75, 76]. The subset of missed lesions that could not be seen despite focused search on second look suggests that truly invisible lesions do exist.

A recent meta-analysis of seven studies including 526 patients showed a pooled sensitivity of 74% for mpMRI in the detection of clinically important cancers [77]. When compared with the current paradigm of PSA measurement and TRUSgBX, the introduction of mpMRI is clearly an improvement. It has recently been demonstrated in a prior cohort study by Ahmed et al. [78], that using mpMRI, allows 27% of patients to avoid a primary biopsy and diagnosis of 5% fewer clinically non-csPCa; and if subsequent TRUSgBX were directed by mpMRI findings, more cases of csPCa might be detected compare to the standard pathway of TRUSgBX for all [78]. This approach could potentially save a quarter of the population from the cost and complications of TRUSgBX. Rosenkrantz et al. [79] showed that mpMRI had a sensitivity of 76% when compared with matched pathology specimens. Similar studies by Le et al. [80] and Russo et al. [81] using pathology results as the reference standard showed 80–90% sensitivity. However, they found that 30% of tumors with a GS > 7 and larger than 1.0 cm were missed at MR imaging [80]. De Visschere et al. [82] reported that the majority of missed lesions were low grade and confined to the organ. A retrospective review of mpMRI in patients with missed lesions in their study revealed that the majority of missed lesions had a lower score, and PCa was multifocal in these patients. A paired analysis in patients in whom prospective reading missed lesions revealed that missed lesions were two to three times smaller in volume (0.86 mL vs. 2.13 mL, P = 0.001), which can be possibly explained by limitations associated with spatial resolution of MR imaging. [75, 82]

5. Conclusion

In conclusion, mpMRI has become an important factor for patients being enrolled in active surveillance protocols for the management of low-grade PCa. mpMRI is a proven imaging modality that can accurately detect csPCa. Several pitfalls, both interpretive and technical, may be encountered at mpMRI of the prostate, and a failure to recognize these pitfalls can lead to suboptimal patient care. Targeted biopsies of mpMRI detected lesions pose a challenge in clinical practice. The limitations of TRUSgBX should be acknowledged in order to improve the diagnostic accuracy of targeted biopsies and finally a detailed understanding of these mpMRI pitfalls is critical for the MR practitioner involved in the management of PCa.

Author details

Alireza Ziaei

Address all correspondence to: aziaei@bwh.harvard.edu

Harvard Medical School, Brigham and Women's Hospital, Boston, USA

References

[1] American Cancer Society. Cancer Facts & Figures 2016. Atlanta: American Cancer Society; 2016

[2] Boesen L. Multiparametric MRI in detection and staging of prostate cancer. Danish Medical Bulletin (online). 2017;**64**(2)

[3] Jemal A, Siegel R, Ward E, Murray T, Xu J, Smigal C, Thun MJ. Cancer statistics, 2006. CA: a Cancer Journal for Clinicians. 2006;**56**(2):106-130

[4] Deongchamps BN, Singh A, Haas GP. Epidemiology of prostate cancer in African: Another step in the understanding of the disease? Current Problems in Cancer. 2007;**31**(3):226-236

[5] Sakr WA, Haas GP, Cassin BF, Pontes JE, Crissman JD. The frequency of carcinoma and intraepithelial neoplasia of the prostate in young male patients. The Journal of Urology. 1993;**150**(2 Pt 1):379-385

[6] Miller KD, Siegel RL, Lin CC, et al. Cancer treatment and survivorship statistics, 2016. CA: a Cancer Journal for Clinicians. 2016;**66**(4):271-289

[7] Loeb S, Bjurlin MA, Nicholson J, et al. Overdiagnosis and overtreatment of prostate cancer. European Urology. 2014;**65**(6):1046-1055

[8] Etzioni R, Penson DF, Legler JM, Di Tommaso D, Boer R, Gann PH, Feuer EJ. Overdiagnosis due to prostate-specific antigen screening: Lessons from US prostate cancer incidence trends. Journal of the National Cancer Institute. 2002 Jul 3;**94**(13):981-990

[9] Wolters T, Roobol MJ, van Leeuwen PJ, et al. A critical analysis of the tumor volume threshold for clinically insignificant prostate cancer using a data set of a randomized screening trial. The Journal of Urology. 2011;**185**(1):121-125

[10] National Comprehensive Cancer Network (NCCN). Clinical practice guidelines in oncology: prostate cancer. Fort Washington, PA; 2012. Available via http://www.nccn.com/files/cancer-guidelines/prostate/index.html#/1. [Accessed Sept. 13, 2013]

[11] Prostate Cancer Canada. Prostate cancer Canada network. Toronto, ON Canada; 2014. Available via http://prostatecancer.ca. [Accessed Sept. 2014]

[12] Potosky AL, Miller BA, Albertsen PC, Kramer BS. The role of increasing detection in the rising incidence of prostate cancer. Journal of the American Medical Association. 1995;**273**(7):548-552

[13] Armenian HK, Lilienfeld AM, Diamond EL, Bross ID. Relation between benign prostatic hyperplasia and cancer of the prostate. A prospective and retrospective study. Lancet. 1974;**2**(7873):115-117

[14] Bostwick DG, Cooner WH, Denis L, Jones GW, Scardino PT, Murphy GP. The association of benign prostatic hyperplasia and cancer of the prostate. Cancer. 1992;**70** (1 Suppl):291-301

[15] Hernández J, Thompson IM. Prostate-specific antigen: A review of the validation of the most commonly used cancer biomarker. Cancer. 2004;**101**:894-904

[16] Thompson IM, Pauler DK, Goodman PJ, Tangen CM, Lucia MS, Parnes HL, et al. Prevalence of prostate cancer among men with a prostate-specific antigen level < or = 4.0 ng per milliliter. The New England Journal of Medicine. 2004;**350**:2239-2246

[17] Catalona WJ, Hudson MA, Scardino PT, Richie JP, Ahmann FR, Flanigan RC, et al. Selection of optimal prostate specific antigen cutoffs for early detection of prostate cancer: Receiver operating characteristic curves. The Journal of Urology. 1994;**152**:2037-2042

[18] De Angelis G, Rittenhouse HG, Mikolajczyk SD, Blair Shamel L, Semjonow A. Twenty years of psa: From prostate antigen to tumor marker. Revista de Urología. 2007;**9**:113-123

[19] Djavan B, Ravery V, Zlotta A, Dobronski P, Dobrovits M, Fakhari M, et al. Prospective evaluation of prostate cancer detected on biopsies 1, 2, 3 and 4: When should we stop? The Journal of Urology. 2001;**166**:1679-1683

[20] Obort AS, Ajadi MB, Akinloye O. Prostate-specific antigen: Any successor in sight? Revista de Urología. 2013;**15**:97-107

[21] Carvalhal GF, Smith DS, Mager DE, Ramos C, Catalona WJ. Digital rectal examination for detecting prostate cancer at prostate specific antigen levels of 4 ng/ml. Or less. The Journal of Urology. 1999;**161**:835-839

[22] Varenhorst E, Berglund K, Löfman O, Pedersen K. Interobserver variation in assessment of the prostate by digital rectal examination. British Journal of Urology. 1993;**72**:173-176

[23] Chodak GW. Early detection and screening for prostatic cancer. Urology. 1989;**34**:10-12 discussion 46-56

[24] Pedersen KV, Carlsson P, Varenhorst E, Löfman O, Berglund K. Screening for carcinoma of the prostate by digital rectal examination in a randomly selected population. BMJ. 1990;**300**:1041-1044

[25] Catalona WJ, Richie JP, Ahmann FR, Hudson MA, Scardino PT, Flanigan RC, et al. Comparison of digital rectal examination and serum prostate specific antigen in the early detection of prostate cancer: Results of a multicenter clinical trial of 6,630 men. The Journal of Urology. 1994;**151**:1283-1290

[26] Gosselaar C, Roobol MJ, Roemeling S, Schröder FH. The role of the digital rectal examination in subsequent screening visits in the European randomized study of screening for prostate cancer (ERSPC), Rotterdam. European Urology. 2008;**54**:581-588

[27] Okotie OT, Roehl KA, Han M, Loeb S, Gashti SN, Catalona WJ. Characteristics of prostate cancer detected by digital rectal examination only. Urology. 2007;**70**:1117-1120

[28] Heidenreich A, Aus G, Bolla M, Joniau S, Matveev VB, Schmid HP, Zattoni F. EAU guidelines on prostate cancer. Actas urologicas espanolas. Feb 2009;**33**(2):113-126

[29] Harvey CJ, Pilcher J, Richenberg J, Patel U, Frauscher F. Applications of transrectal ultrasound in prostate cancer. The British Journal of Radiology. 2012;**85**(Spec Iss 1):S3-S17

[30] Spajic B, Eupic H, Tomas D, Stimac G, Kruslin B, Kraus O. The incidence of hyperechoic prostate cancer in transrectal ultrasound-guided biopsy specimens. Urology. 2007; **70**:734-737

[31] Quon JS, Moosavi B, Khanna M, Flood TA, Lim CS, Schieda N. False positive and false negative diagnoses of prostate cancer at multi-parametric prostate MRI in active surveillance. Insights into imaging. 2015 Aug 1;**6**(4):449-463

[32] Epstein JI, Feng Z, Trock BJ, Pierorazio PM. Upgrading and downgrading of prostate cancer from biopsy to radical prostatectomy: Incidence and predictive factors using the modified Gleason grading system and factoring in tertiary grades. European Urology. 2012 May 31;**61**(5):1019-1024

[33] Rothwax JT, George AK, Wood BJ, Pinto PA. Multiparametric MRI in biopsy guidance for prostate cancer: Fusion-guided. BioMed Research International. 2014;**2014**:439171. DOI: 10.1155/2014/439171

[34] Schoots IG, Roobol MJ, Nieboer D, Bangma CH, Steyerberg EW, Hunink MM. Magnetic resonance imaging–targeted biopsy may enhance the diagnostic accuracy of significant prostate cancer detection compared to standard transrectal ultrasound-guided biopsy: A systematic review and meta-analysis. European Urology. 2015 Sep 30;**68**(3):438-450

[35] Eskew LA, Bare RL, McCullough DL. Systematic 5 region prostate biopsy is superior to sextant method for diagnosing carcinoma of the prostate. The Journal of Urology. 1997;**157**:199-202. DOI: 10.1016/S0022-5347(01)65322-9

[36] Presti JC Jr, O'Dowd GJ, Miller MC, Mattu R, Veltri RW. Extended peripheral zone biopsy schemes increase cancer detection rates and minimize variance in prostate specific antigen and age related cancer rates: Results of a community multi-practice study. The Journal of Urology. 2003;**169**:125-129. DOI: 10.1016/S0022-5347(05)64051-7

[37] Babaian RJ, Toi A, Kamoi K, et al. A comparative analysis of sextant and an extended 11-core multisite directed biopsy strategy. The Journal of Urology. 2000;**163**:152-157. DOI: 10.1016/S0022-5347(05)67993-1

[38] Noguchi M, Stamey TA, McNeal JE, Yemoto CM. Relationship between systematic biopsies and histological features of 222 radical prostatectomy specimens: Lack of prediction of tumor significance for men with nonpalpable prostate cancer. The Journal of Urology. 2001;**166**:104-109. DOI: 10.1016/S0022-5347(05)66086-7

[39] Bott SR, Young MP, Kellett MJ, Parkinson MC. Anterior prostate cancer: Is it more difficult to diagnose? BJU International. 2002;**89**:886-889

[40] Cooperberg MR, Broering JM, Carroll PR. Time trends and local variation in primary treatment of localized prostate cancer. Journal of Clinical Oncology. 2010;**28**(7):1117-1123

[41] Mols F, Korfage IJ, Vingerhoets AJ, Kil PJ, Coebergh JW, Essink-Bot ML, Van de Poll-Franse LV. Bowel, urinary, and sexual problems among long-term prostate cancer survivors: A population-based study. International Journal of Radiation Oncology, Biology, and Physics. 2009 Jan 1;**73**(1):30-38

[42] Adibi M, Pearle MS, Lotan Y. Cost-effectiveness of standard vs intensive antibiotic regimens for transrectal ultrasonography (TRUS)-guided prostate biopsy prophylaxis. BJU International. 2012;**110**(2 Pt 2)

[43] Taylor AK, Zembower TR, Nadler RB, Scheetz MH, Cashy JP, Bowen D, Murphy AB, Dielubanza E, Schaeffer AJ. Targeted antimicrobial prophylaxis using rectal swab cultures in men undergoing transrectal ultrasound guided prostate biopsy is associated with reduced incidence of postoperative infectious complications and cost of care. The Journal of Urology. 2012 Apr 30;**187**(4):1275-1279

[44] Merchea A, Cullinane DC, Sawyer MD, et al. Esophagogastroduodenoscopy-associated gastrointestinal perforations: A single-center experience. Surgery. 2010;**148**(4):876-880 discussion 881-872

[45] Bournet B, Selves J, Grand D, et al. Endoscopic ultrasound-guided fine-needle aspiration biopsy coupled with a KRAS mutation assay using allelic discrimination improves the diagnosis of pancreatic cancer. Journal of Clinical Gastroenterology. 2015;**49**(1):50-56

[46] Court CM, Ankeny JS, Hou S, Tseng HR, Tomlinson JS. Improving pancreatic cancer diagnosis using circulating tumor cells: Prospects for staging and single-cell analysis. Expert Review of Molecular Diagnostics. Nov 2, 2015;**15**(11):1491-1504

[47] Epstein JI, Allsbrook WC, Amin MB, Egevad LL. The 2005 International Society of Urological Pathology (ISUP) consensus conference on Gleason grading of prostatic carcinoma. The American Journal of Surgical Pathology. 2005;**29**:1228-1242

[48] Gleason DF, Mellinger GT. Prediction of prognosis for prostatic adenocarcinoma by combined histological grading and clinical staging. The Journal of Urology. 1974;**111**:58-64

[49] Epstein JI, Allsbrook WC, Amin MB, Egevad LL. Update on the Gleason grading system for prostate cancer. Urologic Pathologists. 2006;**13**:57-59

[50] Egevad L, Granfors T, Karlberg L, Bergh A, Stattin P. Prognostic value of the Gleason score in prostate cancer. BJU International. 2002;**89**:538-542

[51] Rusthoven CG, Carlson JA, Waxweiler TV, Yeh N, Raben D, Flaig TW, et al. The prognostic significance of Gleason scores in metastatic prostate cancer. Urologic Oncology. 2014;**32**:707-713

[52] Brimo F, Montironi R, Egevad L, Erbersdobler A, Lin DW, Nelson JB, et al. Contemporary grading for prostate cancer: Implications for patient care. European Urology. 2013;**63**:892-901

[53] Pierorazio PM, Walsh PC, Partin AW, Epstein JI. Prognostic Gleason grade grouping: Data based on the modified Gleason scoring system. BJU International. 2013;**111**:753-760

[54] Epstein JI, Feng Z, Trock BJ, Pierorazio PM. Upgrading and downgrading of prostate cancer from biopsy to radical prostatectomy: Incidence and predictive factors using the modified Gleason grading system and factoring in tertiary grades. European Urology. 2012;**61**:1019-1024

[55] Delahunt B, Miller RJ, Srigley JR, Evans AJ, Samaratunga H. Gleason grading: Past, present and future. Histopathology. 2012;**60**:75-86

[56] Sobin L, Gospodarowicz MWC. TNM Classification of Malignant Tumours. Urological Tumours. International Union against Cancer. 7th ed. Wiley-Blackwell: Hoboken, NJ; 2009

[57] Sciarra A, Barentsz J, Bjartell A, Eastham J, Hricak H, Panebianco V, et al. Advances in magnetic resonance imaging: How they are changing the management of prostate cancer. European Urology. 2011;**59**:962-977

[58] Steyn JH, Smith FW. Nuclear magnetic resonance imaging of the prostate. British Journal of Urology. 1982;**54**:726-728

[59] Borre M, Lundorf E, Marcussen N, Langkilde NC, Wolf H. Phased array magnetic resonance imaging for staging clinically localised prostate cancer. Acta Oncologica. 2005;**44**:589-592

[60] Eberhardt SC, Carter S, Casalino DD, et al. ACR appropriateness criteria prostate cacer–pretreatment detection, staging, and surveillance. Journal of the American College of Radiology. 2013;**10**:83-92

[61] Barentsz JO, Richenberg J, Clements R, et al. ESUR prostate MR guidelines 2012. European Radiology. 2012;**22**:746-757

[62] Quon JS, Moosavi B, Khanna M, Flood TA, Lim CS, Schieda N. False positive and false negative diagnoses of prostate cancer at multi-parametric prostate MRI in active surveillance. Insights into imaging. 2015 Aug 1;**6**(4):449-463

[63] Boesen L. Multiparametric MRI in detection and staging of prostate cancer. Scandinavian Journal of Urology. 2015;**49**:25-34

[64] Chabanova E, Balslev I, Logager V, Hansen A, Jakobsen H, Kromann-Andersen B, et al. Prostate cancer: 1.5 T endo-coil dynamic contrast-enhanced MRI and MR spectroscopy--correlation with prostate biopsy and prostatectomy histopathological data. European Journal of Radiology. 2011;**80**:292-296

[65] Barentsz JO, Richenberg J, Clements R, Choyke P, Verma S, Villeirs G, et al. ESUR prostate MR guidelines 2012. European Radiology. 2012;**22**:746-757

[66] Heijmink SWTPJ, Fütterer JJ, Hambrock T, Takahashi S, Scheenen TWJ, Huisman HJ, et al. Prostate cancer: Bodyarray versus endorectal coil MR imaging at 3 T--comparison of image quality, localization, and staging performance. Radiology. 2007;**244**:184-195

[67] Turkbey B, Merino MJ, Gallardo EC, Shah V, Aras O, Bernardo M, et al. Comparison of endorectal coil and nonendorectal coil T2W and diffusion-weighted MRI at 3 tesla for localizing prostate cancer: Correlation with wholemount histopathology. Journal of Magnetic Resonance Imaging. 2014;**39**:1443-1448

[68] Heijmink SWTPJ, Fütterer JJ, Strum SS, Oyen WJG, Frauscher F, Witjes JA, et al. State-of-the-art uroradiologic imaging in the diagnosis of prostate cancer. Acta Oncologica. 2011;**50**(Suppl 1):25-38

[69] Boesen L, Thomsen HS. Magnetic resonance imaging in management of prostate cancer. Ugeskrift for Laeger. 2013;**175**:1630-1633

[70] Hamoen EH, de Rooij M, Witjes JA, Barentsz JO, Rovers MM. Use of the prostate imaging reporting and data system (PI-RADS) for prostate cancer detection with multiparametric magnetic resonance imaging: A diagnostic meta-analysis. European Urology. 2014;**67**:1112-1121. DOI: 10.1016/j.eururo.2014.10.033

[71] de Rooij M, Hamoen EH, Futterer JJ, Barentsz JO, Rovers MM. Accuracy of multiparametric MRI for prostate cancer detection: A meta-analysis. American Journal of Roentgenology. 2014;**202**:343-351. DOI: 10.2214/AJR.13.11046

[72] Hegde JV, Mulkern RV, Panych LP, et al. Multiparametric MRI of prostate cancer: An update on state-of-the-art techniques and their performance in detecting and localizing prostate cancer. Journal of Magnetic Resonance Imaging. 2013;**37**:1035-1054

[73] Schoots IG, Petrides N, Giganti F, et al. Magnetic resonance imaging in active surveillance of prostate cancer: A systematic review. European Urology. 2015;**67**:627-636

[74] Quon JS, Moosavi B, Khanna M, Flood TA, Lim CS, Schieda N. False positive and false negative diagnoses of prostate cancer at multi-parametric prostate MRI in active surveillance. Insights into imaging. 2015 Aug 1;**6**(4):449-463

[75] Borofsky S, George AK, Gaur S, Bernardo M, Greer MD, Mertan FV, Taffel M, Moreno V, Merino MJ, Wood BJ, Pinto PA. What are we missing? False-negative cancers at multiparametric MR imaging of the prostate. Radiology. 2017 Oct;**20**:152877

[76] Vargas HA, Hötker AM, Goldman DA, Moskowitz CS, Gondo T, Matsumoto K, Ehdaie B, Woo S, Fine SW, Reuter VE, Sala E. Updated prostate imaging reporting and data system (PIRADS V2) recommendations for the detection of clinically significant prostate cancer using multiparametric MRI: Critical evaluation using whole-mount pathology as standard of reference. European Radiology. 2016 Jun 1;**26**(6):1606-1612

[77] de Rooij M, Hamoen EH, Fütterer JJ, Barentsz JO, Rovers MM. Accuracy of multiparametric MRI for prostate cancer detection: A meta-analysis. American Journal of Roentgenology. 2014;**202**(2):343-351

[78] Ahmed HU, Bosaily AE, Brown LC, Gabe R, Kaplan R, Parmar MK, Collaco-Moraes Y, Ward K, Hindley RG, Freeman A, Kirkham AP. Diagnostic accuracy of multi-parametric MRI and TRUS biopsy in prostate cancer (PROMIS): A paired validating confirmatory study. The Lancet. 2017 Mar 3;**389**(10071):815-822

[79] Rosenkrantz AB, Deng FM, Kim S, et al. Prostate cancer: multiparametric MRI for index lesion localization: a multiple-reader study. AJR. American Journal of Roentgenology. 2012;**199**(4):830-837

[80] Le JD, Tan N, Shkolyar E, et al. Multifocality and prostate cancer detection by multiparametric magnetic resonance imaging: Correlation with whole-mount histopathology. European Urology. 2015;**67**(3):569-576

[81] Russo F, Regge D, Armando E, et al. Detection of prostate cancer index lesions with multiparametric magnetic resonance imaging (mp-MRI) using whole-mount histological sections as the reference standard. BJU International. 2016;**118**(1):84-94

[82] De Visschere PJ, Naesens L, Libbrecht L, et al. What kind of prostate cancers do we miss on multiparametric magnetic resonance imaging? European Radiology. 2016;**26**(4):1098-1107

Treatment Strategeies

Chapter 3

Advanced Radiation Treatment Planning of Prostate Cancer

Bora Tas

Additional information is available at the end of the chapter

http://dx.doi.org/10.5772/intechopen.76184

Abstract

External beam radiotherapy has been playing a major role in the treatment of prostate cancer with excellent tumor control. Also, localization of prostate is a big challenge for excellent treatment, so we focus on actual IGRT techniques (ultrasound, EMF, etc.) for intrafraction and interfraction motion detection. We investigate several studies related with dose distribution of treatment planning techniques. Several studies have demonstrated the superiority of volumetric modulated arc therapy (VMAT) plans in prostate cancer. We also investigate hypofractionation and stereotactic radiation outcome instead of conventional fractionation for prostate cancer. We mention about prostate cancer's treatment in future by using MR-based linac online adaptive radiotherapy.

Keywords: VMAT, IMRT, IGRT, prostate cancer

1. Introduction

Prostate cancer is one of the most common cancers in the world, and the population of patients with intermediate-to-high-risk localized prostate cancer occupies a large proportion. Most prostate cancers are diagnosed at an early stage, allowing for the high rate of success with localized treatment. Between 30 and 45% of men receive radiation as their primary treatment for prostate cancer depending on their age [1, 2]. External beam radiotherapy (EBRT) and brachytherapy can be used for the treatment of prostate cancer. The differences and roles of these two techniques rely on the physical properties of the radiation and its delivery method. The goal of radiotherapy treatment is to deliver a powerful dose of radiation that will kill the cancer but to do it as precisely as possible so that we cause minimal damage to the healthy tissue such as the urethra, rectum, bladder, and bowel around it. External beam radiotherapy is used as a curative treatment in men with localized prostate cancer (stage T1 or T2) or with locally advanced disease. External beam radiotherapy can also be very helpful to men with advanced prostate cancer. It can ease pain in the bones and reduce the likelihood of having a fracture. Three-dimensional conformal radiotherapy (3DCRT), intensity-modulated radiotherapy (IMRT), and volumetric modulated arc therapy (VMAT) techniques are all applied for this purpose.

2. Treatment planning and image-guided radiotherapy (IGRT) methods

The prostate and seminal vesicles are located between the rectum and the bladder. The position of the prostate is affected by physiologic changes in the bladder and rectum volume. These variations in position and shape can be left unchanged and compensated with margins or reduced by image guidance resulting in smaller irradiated volumes. Smaller margins reduce the dose to the organs at risk; therefore, effort has been directed at reducing uncertainties with the use of image guidance. Radiation oncology has seen a rapid increase in the use of image-guided radiotherapy (IGRT) technology for prostate cancer patients. Conformal high-dose radiotherapy delivered with conventional fractionation results in a significant biochemical control with acceptable toxicities and currently represents the standard therapy when radiotherapy is chosen as primary treatment.

2.1. Three-dimensional conformal radiotherapy (3DCRT) technique

3DCRT uses computed tomography (CT) scanning to plot exact anatomy and to come up with the optimal radiation dosages. 3DCRT can accurately use a patient's unique anatomy to deliver radiation exactly where the patient needs it, while avoiding the bladder, rectum, urethra, and bowel. Conventional 3DCRT treatment planning is manually optimized. This means that the treatment planner chooses all beam parameters, such as the number of beams, beam directions, multileaf collimators (MLCs), shapes, weights, etc., and the computer calculates the resulting dose distribution. 3DCRT in prostate cancer patients is a highly sophisticated and time-consuming method of dose delivery.

2.2. Intensity-modulated radiotherapy (IMRT) technique

In the treatment of prostate cancer, IMRT was introduced in the early 1990s at a number of centers. After advance IGRT methods were implemented to clinic, IMRT technique started to be more popular. IMRT, like 3DCRT, uses high-tech computer software and relies on more than 100 digital CT scans to build a three-dimensional picture of the prostate tumor and organs at risks (OARs), but it can supply even more conformal dose distribution than 3DCRT. We can modulate the intensity of each beam during treatment with a MLC. In the case of IMRT, dose distribution is inversely determined, meaning that the treatment planner has to decide before the dose distribution he wants and the computer then calculates a group of beam intensities that will be produced, as nearly as possible to the desired dose distribution. We can maximize the dose of radiation to the tumor volume and minimize the dose that affects the healthy tissue nearby. With the largest experience being detailed at the Memorial Sloan Kettering Cancer Center. Zelefsky et al. [3] reported on the treatment of 1571 patients with IMRT at doses as high as 81 Gy, with rates of gastrointestinal (GI) and genitourinary (GU) toxicity less than those reported from their institution for 3DCRT at similar or lower doses. Likewise, Kupelian et al. [4] reported results on a large study involving 770 patients treated at the Cleveland Clinic with intensity-modulated techniques at biologically effective doses comparable with those at the Memorial Sloan Kettering Cancer Center and with similar low rates of GI and GU toxicity. This means less collateral damage to noncancerous tissue that's just minding its own business right next to the tumor in the bladder and rectum and fewer side effects.

2.3. Volumetric modulated arc therapy (VMAT) technique

Volumetric modulated arc therapy (VMAT) has attracted increasing attention because of its greatly improved delivery efficiency over fixed-field IMRT. Unlike IMRT, which typically includes less than 10 fixed-field beam angles, VMAT includes a large number of beam directions from an arc trajectory and delivers doses dynamically during rotation of the gantry.

VMAT is a novel radiation technique, which can achieve highly conformal dose distributions with improved target volume coverage and sparing of normal tissues compared with conventional radiotherapy techniques. VMAT also has the potential to offer additional advantages, such as reduced treatment delivery time compared with conventional static-field IMRT. The clinical worldwide use of VMAT is increasing significantly [5].

3DCRT was incapable of covering a modern radiotherapy volume for the radical treatment of prostate cancer. These volumes can be treated via conventional IMRT and VMAT. VMAT was

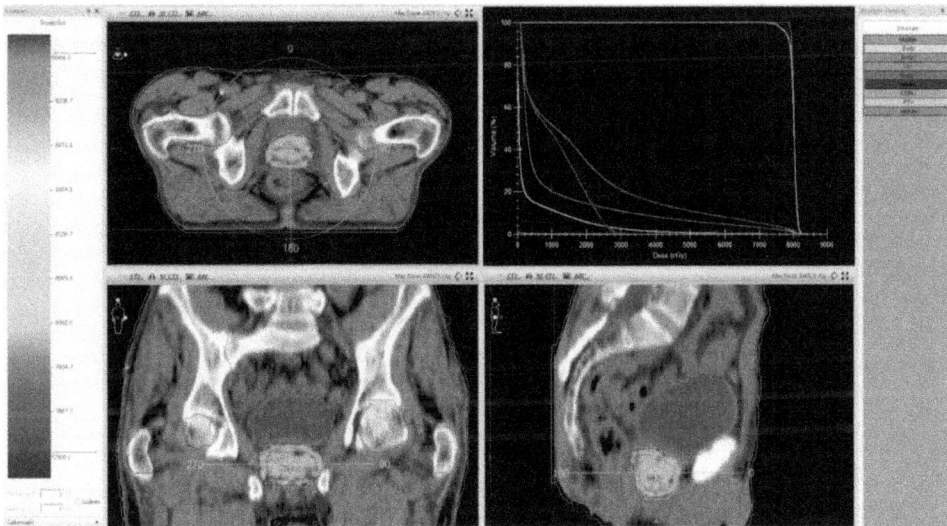

Figure 1. Dose distribution of prostate cancer treatment planning by using VMAT technique.

significantly more efficient than IMRT. VMAT technologies are a superior way of delivering IMRT treatments [6]. VMAT treatment plan is shown in **Figure 1**.

VMAT has slightly better CI, while the volume of low doses was higher. VMAT had lower MUs than IMRT. VMAT can shorten room times and improve patient throughput over seven-field DMLC IMRT.

2.4. Image-guided radiotherapy (IGRT) methods

Radiation oncology has seen a rapid increase in the use of image-guided radiotherapy (IGRT) technology for prostate cancer patients over the past decade. Prostate can move around in there by as much as a centimeter, depending on how full your bladder and rectum are. IGRT approach has a lot of flexibility, because the radiation oncologist uses CT scan images to point the exact location of the prostate each day.

Perirectal sparing with placement biomaterials between the posterior prostate and the anterior rectum has shown promise in reducing the radiation dose received by the rectal wall when used in the setting of conventional fractionated radiotherapy [7, 8]. Perirectal sparing biomaterials may promote not only sparing of the rectum wall but also result in decreased dose to other organs at risk including the penile bulb and bladder (**Figure 2**).

Linear accelerators equipped with kilovoltage (kV) cone-beam computed tomography (CBCT) allow for soft tissue registration immediately before treatment over the past decade [9]. Image guidance was either by implanted fiducials and daily kilovoltage imaging or with the use of cone-beam computed tomography (CBCT). IGRT is an excellent method for dose-escalated external beam radiotherapy in the treatment of localized prostate cancer in regard to GU and GI toxicity (**Figure 3**).

It is well documented that the prostate bed is highly susceptible to inter-fraction motion leading to larger treatment planning margins to account for daily treatment setup uncertainties when matching bony anatomy. Organ motion can be a significant barrier to delivering accurate external beam radiotherapy to the prostate. The use of fiducial markers in the prostate bed has significantly improved the accuracy of the treatment delivery.

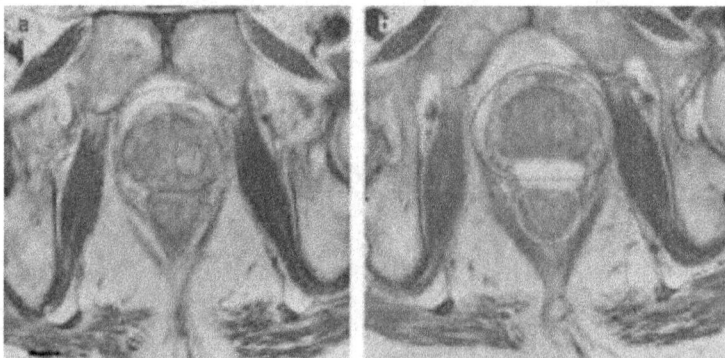

Figure 2. MR images of perirectal sparing with biomaterials and without it.

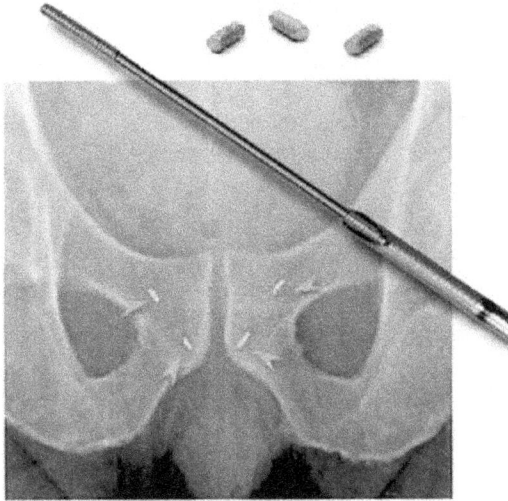

Figure 3. Fiducial markers image.

With CBCT scan-based correction strategies, one should be able to overcome the limitations of marker-based strategies. Smitsmans et al. [10] developed an automatic, rigid, three-dimensional (3D) gray-value registration (3D-GR) method for fast prostate localization on CT scans. In a following study, they showed that the 3D-GR prostate localization also worked with CBCT scans and concluded that CBCT scans could be used for image-guided radiotherapy for prostate cancer [11]. Using the daily CBCT scans, we could compare today's images with yesterday's and tune the treatment accordingly. Many studies have been reported on image guidance strategies to correct for prostate motion with daily offline or online position verification of the prostate. Most of these reports used implanted fiducial markers in the prostate [12, 13]. Although fiducial marker-based correction strategies are already an important step forward, they have some shortcomings. The implantation of markers is an invasive procedure. Marker-based strategies correct for translations but tend to neglect rotations, which are known to be a large component of prostate motion [14]. Also, marker-based correction strategies do not take into account changes in position of the seminal vesicles or the effect of a changed anatomy on planning, especially relevant for IMRT.

The Calypso® (Varian Medical Systems, Palo Alto, USA) system uses radio-frequency waves that allow very accurate alignment of the prostate before each treatment session and at all times during treatment delivery. The Calypso® system improves the ability to target radiation only to tumor volume, avoiding unnecessary radiation to healthy tissues such as the bladder and rectum. The Calypso localization and tracking system works with three Beacon® transponders, wireless electromagnetic circuits about the size of a grain of rice, that are implanted in the prostate. It is shown in **Figure 4**. The Calypso® system works with the transponders to locate the tumor's position, guide the therapist to set up the treatment continuously through radiotherapy, and tailor treatment delivery to trigger the beam on and off to ensure the tumor is accurately aligned throughout the treatment [15]. In addition, the data demonstrate that treatment with VMAT permits the use of advanced prostate tracking (Calypso®), resulting in similar treatment times as standard seven-field

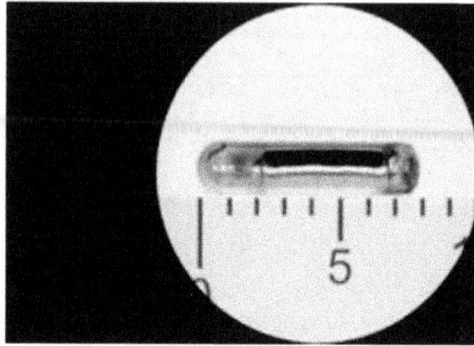

Figure 4. A Beacon® transponder.

dynamic multileaf collimator (DMLC) IMRT with conventional tracking [16]. Foster et al. [17] determined the differences between CBCT-Calypso® and kV imaging-Calypso® localizations are 0.31 ± 1.82, 0.00 ± 1.00, and − 028 ± 1.36 and 0.28 ± 4.12, −0.28 ± 3.22, and 0.16 ± 1.61 mm, respectively, in the AP, SI, and RL directions during 160 and 100 fractions each These results show good localization agreement between radiographic technique and electromagnetic transponder technique, indicating that each of the localization technique is suitable for prostate cancer.

The functionality of RayPilot® (Micropos Medical, Sweden) is similar to a GPS by means that a target is localized with given coordinates. The system communicates with an implanted transmitter that is located in the ROI to be treated. The transmitter sends signals to a sensor plate 30 times per second, and the position is presented in the software. The system consists of the RayPilot® receiving system which is placed on any existing treatment couch, the RayPilot transmitter that is placed in the ROI, and the RayPilot® software. Initially, the system is used in treatment of prostate cancer as IGRT system [18].

Noninvasive 4D transperineal ultrasound (4D-TPUS) has been introduced in tracking intrafractional prostate motion in radiotherapy. Compared to other tracking methods, the ultrasound has its own advantage in precise identification of the soft tissue without invasive procedure or extra radiation dose. In addition, system supplies contouring tool for prostate and OAR volume while doing CT/ultrasound image fusion in the same patient position. Clarity® (Elekta AB, Stockholm, Sweden) 4D monitoring during prostate treatment offers live imaging of the target and surrounding anatomy. The target position is automatically calculated and compared to physician action thresholds to enable intrafraction motion management (**Figure 5**).

Ultrasound provides real-time position data for the prostate that was used to gate the treatment. Ultrasound motion data provides margin guidelines for clinics without ultrasound that treat prostate SBRT with a rectal balloon, based on their expected treatment length and acceptable probability of prostate excursion beyond margins. Qi et al. [19] determined the median (5–95% percentile) of 221 intrafraction prostate motions in the L−/R+, S+/I−, and A+/P− were 0.1 mm (−1.13 to 1.64 mm), −0.1 mm (−1.89 to 1.90 mm), and − 0.3 mm (−2.88 to 1.25 mm) by using 4D-TPUS. There were 70/221 (32%) fractions with deviation exceeding 2 mm in any direction, with an average duration of 26% of treatment time, while there were 19/221 (8.6%)

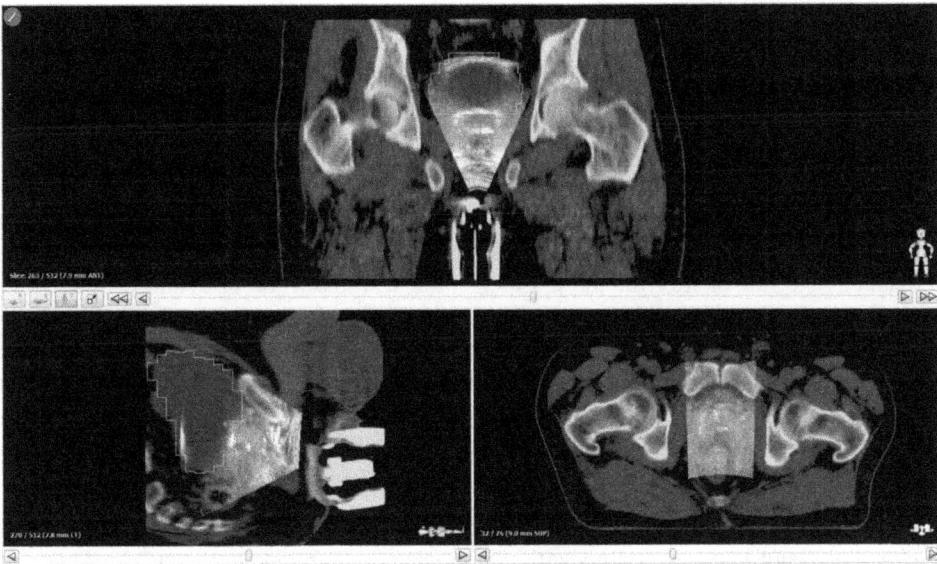

Figure 5. Image fusion between CT and ultrasound.

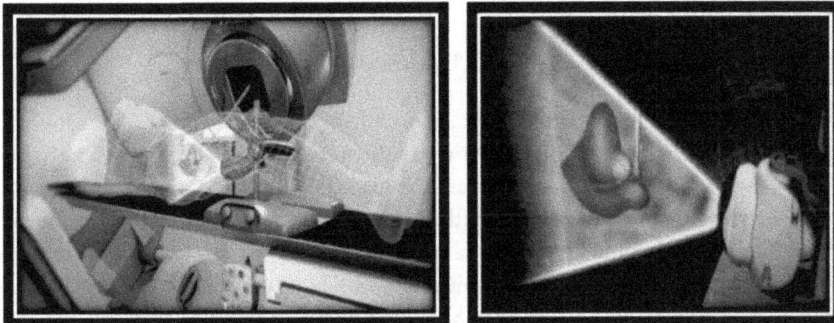

Figure 6. 4D transperineal ultrasound scanning.

fractions with deviation exceeding 3 mm in any direction with an average duration of 6.3% of treatment time. These data can help to understand the intrafraction motion of the prostate and may allow a reduction of treatment margin (**Figure 6**).

2.5. Hypofractionation radiotherapy technique

Many studies have shown a lower α/β value (1.4–3.1 Gy) for prostate cancer than most of other cancers. This indicates that prostate cancer would be more responsive to the size of fractional dose rather than the total dose. Due to this radiobiological feature, the hypothesis is that hypofractionation would yield non-inferior or even better local control than conventional fractionated radiotherapy without increasing the risk of treatment-related toxicities. A series of equivalent hypofractionation regimens suitable for the IMRT simultaneous integrated boost (SIB) were obtained for high-risk prostate cancer. For example, the conventional treatment regimen of 42 × 1.8 Gy (EUD = 75.4 Gy) would be equivalent to a SIB regimen of 25 × 2.54 Gy. Compared to the conventional two-phase treatment, the proposed SIB technique offers potential advantages, including better sparing of critical structures, more efficient delivery, shorter treatment duration, and better biological effectiveness for high-risk prostate cancer treatment [20].

Hypofractionated image-guided radiotherapy with 15 fractions of 3.65 Gy/3 weeks is well tolerated with a low rate of acute and late grade ≥ 2 GI and GU toxicities. This schedule permits to obtain a high rate of survival and disease control with reduction of treatment time spent for treatment by patients [21]. Hypofractionated intensity-modulated radiotherapy of 45 Gy in nine consecutive fractions' regime for mainly low−/intermediate-risk prostate cancer patients is favorable with low rates of late toxicity [22]. Hypofractionated radiotherapy with IMRT-IGRT as primary treatment for prostate cancer allows reduction in overall treatment time without compromising outcomes. This Hypo-IMRT with IGRT schedule for prostate radiotherapy reduces treatment length by 2 weeks as compared to the other treatment regimens commonly used.

Compared with conventional radiotherapy, hypofractionated radiotherapy has achieved similar clinical outcomes in patients with intermediate-to-high-risk localized PCa. Although hypofractionated radiotherapy has an increased incidence rate of acute gastrointestinal adverse events, the late gastrointestinal and genitourinary adverse events were similar in two groups and could be tolerable for the patients.

2.6. Stereotactic body radiotherapy (SBRT) technique

Stereotactic body radiotherapy (SBRT) is an established treatment technique for prostate cancer. High dose per fraction radiotherapy has theoretical advantages when treating "late responding tissue." SBRT for high-risk prostate cancer (PCa) remains investigational not only due to concerns for potential toxicity when the treatment volumes extend beyond the prostate gland itself. Specifically, some investigators have reported high rates of toxicity when targeting elective pelvic nodal irradiation volumes with SBRT techniques, but technical considerations may have influenced those results. SBRT regimes can be safely used to treat patients with high-risk PCa in a total of 5 treatment days. The addition of pelvic nodal radiation did not significantly increase acute or late genitourinary or gastrointestinal toxicity on either physician- or patient-reported scales [23].

Dose escalation beyond currently standard SBRT regimens may further improve outcomes, particularly for bulkier tumors, but could be limited by organ dose constraints. However, selective dose escalation to identified regions of high tumor burden may offer a safer approach than uniform dose escalation, thereby maximizing therapeutic ratio. Therefore, this ongoing prospective study seeks to test the planning and delivery feasibilities and the tolerability of treating patients with a modest dose escalation to the entire prostate and a SIB to magnetic resonance (MR)-identified lesions (**Figure 7**).

Chapet et al. [24] compared acute toxicities of moderate hypofractionation versus stereotactic radiation for prostate cancer. They determined that hypofractionation and SBRT are well tolerated in only two grade 3 acute GU toxicities and only one grade 3 GI toxicity. There is no

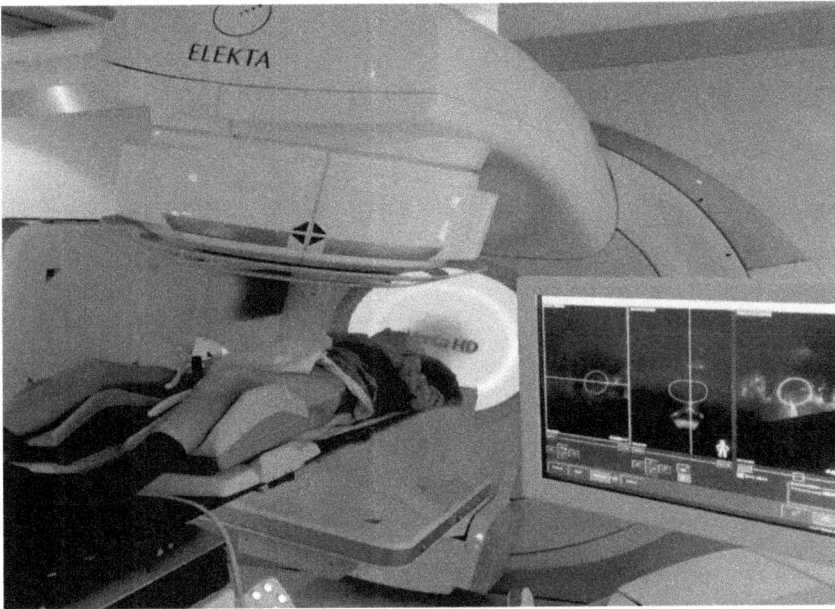

Figure 7. Prostate SBRT treatment by using 4D TPUS Clarity® IGRT system and versa HD® linear accelerator.

difference in grade ≥ 2 acute toxicities, the acute profile of tolerance appears to be the same between hypofractionation and SBRT for urinary toxicities, and acute GI toxicities seem to be well controlled by the spacer whatever fractionation is used.

SBRT for prostate cancer has become increasingly popular, but the use of hypofraction-ation necessitates special consideration of the normal tissue tolerances of organs such as the urethra, bladder, and rectum. Tracking prostatic motion in real time provides more precise treatment by allowing a repositioning of the treatment couch if the fiducials move outside a threshold margin. Although soft tissue anatomy is not readily visualized in real time during treatment, fiducial marker position is used as a surrogate for target/organ-at-risk geometry. Because of the observed random distribution of motion, we hypothesize that CBCT's performed before and after treatment may miss intrafraction movements that exceed the threshold margin. Due to intrafractional movement, positioning the patient exclusively based on the pretreatment CBCT scans is insufficient to ensure complete target coverage. Intrafractional on-demand imaging is required to ensure adequate coverage to the PTV.

Robotic SBRT of soft tissue lesions using Cyberknife® (Accuray, Sunnyvale, USA) requires implantation of fiducial markers for target tracking by the stereoscopic KV X-ray imaging system. The spatial distribution of the fiducials must allow accurate calculation of 3D transformation that describes the position of the prostate within the reference frame of the planning CT scan. Poor fiducial placement limits accurate tracking. Creating fiducial implantation protocol could improve ability to accurately track prostate motion during treatment. In order to take into account intrafraction rotation, a minimal spacing of 1.8 cm must be achieved between

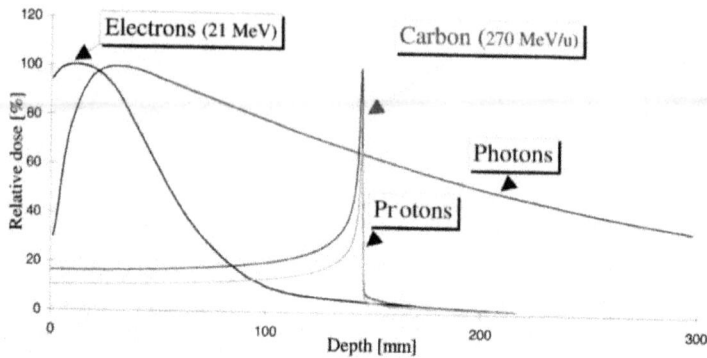

Figure 8. Depth dose curves of electron, photon, proton, and carbon beams.

implanted markers. This is frequently accomplished with double-loaded needles with spacers present or rigidly attached to the markers.

Advanced IGRT methods such as ultrasound, EMF, etc. with perirectal sparing biomaterials and/or fiducial markers can supply significantly advantage for accurate hypofractionation and SBRT treatment of prostate cancer.

Protons have completely different dose distribution properties and have the potential to avoid most of the extra-target radiation that is inherent to photons. Unlike a photon, a proton is a heavy particle (roughly 1800 times the mass of an electron) with an elementary charge, which confers certain dosimetric advantages. Heavy particles, as opposed to photons, will stop within a target. This unique property allows protons to be targeted so that they have their most damaging effects in the tumor itself, with less radiation delivered in front of the target, and no dose delivered beyond it. This peak of energy delivery is commonly referred to as the Bragg peak. It is shown in **Figure 8**. The Bragg peak is very narrow and must be spread out using multiple proton energies to ensure that the peak encompasses the entire target.

Proton beam therapy for prostate cancer has become a source of controversy in the urologic community, and the rapid dissemination and marketing of this technology have led to many patients inquiring about this therapy. Several groups [25–30] have investigated the dosimetric quality of proton therapy for prostate cancer. Rana et al. [31] determined the average differ-ence in the PTV doses between the VMAT and lateral two-field proton plans was within ±1%. On average, the proton plans produced a lower mean dose to the rectum (18.2 Gy (relative biological effectiveness [RBE]) vs. 40.0 Gy) and bladder (15.8 Gy (RBE) vs. 30.1 Gy), whereas the mean dose to the femoral heads was lower in the VMAT plans (28.3 Gy (RBE) vs. 19.3 Gy).

Magnetic resonance images (MRI) demonstrate superior soft tissue contrast such as the pros-tate, rectum, bladder, etc. than CT scans. MR based-linac offers a clinically proven on-table MRI-guided online adaptive, automated and integrated treatment planning system that uses a linac to deliver modulated radiotherapy. Magnetic resonance radiotherapy (MR/RT) system is capable of delivering precisely targeted radiation doses while simultaneously captur-ing magnetic resonance (MR) images. We expect significantly decreased target margin and increased target dosage by using online adaptive MRI-based linac in the future (**Figure 9**).

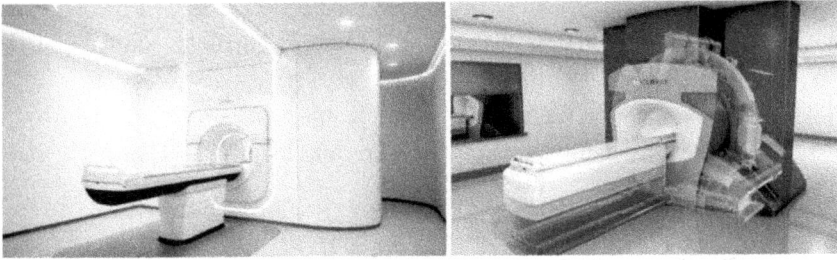

Figure 9. MR-based linac Elekta Unity® and ViewRay® MRIdian.

Author details

Bora Tas

Address all correspondence to: bora_tash@yahoo.com

Department of Radiation Oncology, Yeni Yuzyil University Gaziosmanpasa Hospital,
Istanbul, Turkey

References

[1] Meltzer D, Egleston B, Abdalla I. Patterns of prostate cancer treatment by clinical stage and age. American Journal of Public Health. 2001;**91**(1):126-128

[2] Dinan MA, Robinson TJ, Zagar TM, et al. Changes in initial treatment for prostate cancer among Medicare beneficiaries, 1999-2007. International Journal of Radiation Oncology, Biology, Physics. 2012;**82**(5):e781-e786

[3] Zelefsky MJ, Levin EJ, Hunt M, et al. Incidence of late rectal and urinary toxicities after three-dimensional conformal radiotherapy and intensity-modulated radiotherapy for localized prostate cancer. International Journal of Radiation Oncology, Biology, Physics. 2008;**70**(4):1124e1129

[4] Kupelian PA, Willoughby TR, Reddy CA, Klein EA, Mahadevan A. Hypofractionated intensity-modulated radiotherapy (70 Gy at 2.5 Gy per fraction) for localized prostate cancer: Cleveland Clinic experience. International Journal of Radiation Oncology, Biology, Physics. 2007;**68**(5):1424-1430

[5] Teoh M, Clark CH, Wood K, Whitaker S, Nisbet A, Volumetric modulated arc therapy: A review of current literature and clinical use in practice. British Journal of Radiology. 2011;**84**(1007):967-996

[6] Gerald BF, Diana Ng, Guilin L, Lauren EH, Nastik B. Volumetric modulated arc therapy is superior to conventional intensity modulated radiotherapy – A comparison among prostate cancer patients treated in an Australian Centre, Radiation Oncology; 2011;**6**:108

[7]   Hamstra A, Mariados N, Sylevter J, et al. Continued benefit to rectal separation for prostate radiation therapy: Final results of phase III trial. International Journal of Radiation Oncology, Biology, Physics 2017;**97**(5):976-985

[8]   Pinkawa M, Berneking V, Schlenter M, et al. Quality of life after radiation therapy for prostate cancer with a hydrogel spacer: 5-year results. International Journal of Radiation Oncology, Biology, Physics. 2017;**99**(2):374-377

[9]   Jaffray DA, Siewerdsen JH. Cone-beam computed tomography with flat-panel imager: Initial performance characterization. Medical Physics. 2000;**27**:1311-1323

[10] Smitsmans MH, Wolthaus JWH, Artignan X, et al. Automatic localization of the prostate for on-line or off-line image-guided radiotherapy. International Journal of Radiation Oncology, Biology, Physics. 2004;**60**:623-635

[11] Smitsmans MHP, De Bois J, Sonke JJ, et al. Automatic prostate localization on cone-beam CT scans for high precision image-guided radiotherapy. International Journal of Radiation Oncology, Biology, Physics. 2005;**63**:975-984

[12] Van den Heuvel F, Fugazzi J, Seppi E, et al. Clinical application of a repositioning scheme, using gold markers and electronic portal imaging. Radiotherapy and Oncology. 2006;**79**:94-100

[13] Litzenberg DW, Balter JM, Hadley SW, et al. Influence of intrafraction motion on margins for prostate radiotherapy. International Journal of Radiation Oncology, Biology, Physics. 2006;**65**:548-553

[14] Hoogeman MS, van Herk M, de Bois J, et al. Strategies to reduce the systematic error due to tumor and rectum motion in radiotherapy of prostate cancer. Radiotherapy and Oncology. 2005;**74**:177-185

[15] Virginia Mason Medical Centre. March 2018. Retrieved from: https://www.virginiamason.org/prostate-cancer-calypso-system

[16] William AH, Timothy HF, Xiaojun J, Roshan SP, Peter JR, Karen G, Ashesh BJ. Treatment efficiency of volumetric modulated arc therapy in comparison with intensity-modulated radiotherapy in the treatment of prostate cancer. Journal of the American College of Radiology. 2013;**10**(2):128-134

[17] Foster RD, Papiez E, Solberg TD. Comparison of localization techniques for prostate radiotherapy. In: World Congress on Medical Physics and Biomedical Engineering, September 7-12, 2009, Munich, Germany. pp 784-787

[18] Micropos Medical (n.d.). November 2017. Retrieved from: https://www.micropos.se/products/

[19] Qi X, Gao XS, Yu H, Qin SB, Li HZ. Real-time prostate tracking in prostate cancer radiotherapy using autoscan transperineal ultrasound, ESTRO 35 2016, PO-0879. Radiation & Oncology. April, 2016;**119**(1):S421-422

[20] Li XA, Wang JZ, Jursinic PA, Lawton CA, Wang D. Dosimetric advantages of IMRT simultaneous integrated boost for high risk prostate cancer. International Journal of Radiation Oncology, Biology, Physics. Mar 15, 2005;**61**(4):1251-1257

[21] Bonome P, Osti MF, Giuliani M, De Sanctis V, Cavivano D, Valeriani M. Intermediate risk prostate cancer patients treated with image guided hypofractionated radiation therapy, Astro. International Journal of Radiation Oncology, Biology, Physics. October 1, 2017;**99**(2):E216

[22] Liu Y, Jing J, Wang S, Dai J, Li Y. Evaluation of a hypofractionated intensity modulated radiation therapy schema (45 Gy at 5Gy per fraction) in the treatment of localized prostate cancer, Astro. International Journal of Radiation Oncology, Biology, Physics. October 1, 2017;**99**(2):E252-253

[23] Kishan AU, Fuller DB, Steinberg ML, Ramirez V, Ostendorf E, Tsai S et al., Stereotactic body radiotherapy for high risk prostate cancer: Preliminary toxicity results of phase II trial. Astro. International Journal of Radiation Oncology, Biology, Physics. October 1, 2017;**99**(2):E248

[24] Chapet O, Laroche GD, BIN S, Latorzeff I, Supiot S, Votron L et al. Prostate hypofractionated radiotherapy with a rectal spacer comparing moderate hypofractionation (62 Gy at 3.1 Gy per fraction) versus stereotactic irradiation (37.5 Gy at 7.5 Gy per fraction) acute toxicities from the rpah2 randomized trial. Astro. International Journal of Radiation Oncology, Biology, Physics. October 1, 2017;**99**(2):E218-219

[25] Chera BS, Vargas C, Morris CG, Louis D, Flampouri S, Yeung D, Duvvuri S, Li Z, Mendenhall NP. Dosimetric study of pelvic proton radiotherapy for high-risk prostate cancer. International Journal of Radiation Oncology, Biology, Physics. 2009;**75**:994-1002

[26] Fontenot JD, Lee AK, Newhauser WD. Risk of secondary malignant neoplasms from proton therapy and intensity-modulated X-ray therapy for early-stage prostate cancer. International Journal of Radiation Oncology, Biology, Physics. 2009;**74**:616-622

[27] Zhang X, Dong L, Lee AK, Cox JD, Kuban DA, Zhu RX, Wang X, Li Y, Newhauser WD, Gillin M, Mohan R. Effect of anatomic motion on proton therapy dose distributions in prostate cancer treatment. International Journal of Radiation Oncology, Biology, Physics. 2007;**67**:620-629

[28] Nihei K, Ogino T, Onozawa M, Murayama S, Fuji H, Murakami M, Hishikawa Y. Multiinstitutional phase II study of proton beam therapy for organ-confined prostate cancer focusing on the incidence of late rectal toxicities. International Journal of Radiation Oncology, Biology, Physics. 2011;**81**:390-396

[29] Soukup M, Sohn M, Yan D, Liang J, Alber M. Study of robustness of IMPT and IMRT for prostate cancer against organ movement. International Journal of Radiation Oncology, Biology, Physics. 2009;**75**:941-949

[30] Vargas C, Fryer A, Mahajan C, Indelicato D, Horne D, Chellini A, McKenzie C, Lawlor P, Henderson R, Li Z, Lin L, Olivier K, Keole S. Dose-volume comparison of proton therapy and intensity-modulated radiotherapy for prostate cancer. International Journal of Radiation Oncology, Biology, Physics. 2008;**70**:744-751

[31] Rana S, Cheng CY, Zheng Y, Risalvato D, Cersonsky N, Ramirez E, et al. Proton therapy vs. VMAT for prostate cancer: A treatment planning study. International Journal of Particle Therapy. Apr 2014;**1**(1):22-33

Chapter 4

Role of miR-2909 in Prostate Carcinogenesis

Shiekh Gazalla Ayub

Additional information is available at the end of the chapter

http://dx.doi.org/10.5772/intechopen.76372

Abstract

The biggest challenge in prostate cancer treatment is to understand the signaling mechanisms controlling disease progression. In this context, microRNAs assume huge importance and have recently become an attractive area of research. MicroRNAs are naturally occurring, single-stranded, small non-coding RNAs of 19–25 nucleotides that regulate gene expression. MicroRNAs function as oncogenes or tumor-suppressor genes, and their deregulation is a common feature of human cancers including prostate cancer. Among deregulated microRNAs in prostate cancer, some microRNAs are directly under androgen receptor signaling control and function as the effectors of androgen signaling. Recent findings have shown that apoptosis antagonizing transcription factor (AATF) gene encodes a microRNA designated as miR-2909 that plays an important role in prostate cancer progression. miR-2909 is identified as an androgen-regulated microRNA acting as a novel effector of androgen/androgen receptor signaling. It enhances the proliferation potential of prostate cancer cells and assists in prostate cancer survival under reduced androgen levels by maintaining a positive feedback loop with AR. miR-2909 exerts its oncogenic effects via multiple mechanisms including attenuation of tumor-suppressive effects of TGFβ signaling by directly targeting TGFBR2 and via STAT1 pathway and upregulation of ISGylation pathway through SOCS3/STAT1 pathway.

Keywords: prostate cancer, hormone-sensitive, castration-resistant, androgen receptor, TGFβ, TGFBR2, ISG15, SOCS3, STAT1

1. Introduction

Cancer is one of the leading causes of deaths at the global level accounting for 8.2 million deaths in 2012 [1]. Among males, prostate gland is one of the five leading sites of cancer accounting for approximately 15% of cancers in men, and the incidence is expected to rise steeply by around 19% in the coming years [2, 3]. Prostate cancer (PCa) causes substantial clinical, social and economical burden in both the developing and developed world. The prostate specific antigen (PSA), a protein mainly secreted by prostate cells, is a blood-based marker routinely used for early-stage PCa detection as well as to monitor recurrence of PCa after initial treatment [4]. Even though PSA is a valuable tool, it lacks specificity and is therefore not considered an optimal biomarker [5]. Thus, additional novel biomarkers are needed which can help to predict the exact level of disease aggressiveness, assist in clinical decision about the choice of treatment and aid in establishing more persuasive treatment for the advanced PCa. Prostate tumors are reported to display novel recurrent chromosomal translocations and aberrant expressions of certain microRNAs (miRNAs) which can be helpful for elucidating PCa biology and explored for better disease management [6]. Identification of dysregulated genes or miRNAs in PCa cannot only be promising in terms of diagnostics and therapeutics but can provide clues relevant to disease etiology and progression. miRNAs are small noncoding RNAs that finely regulate gene expression in cells. Alterations in miRNA expression have been reported to be associated with PCa development and are currently being thoroughly investigated as PCa biomarkers. Several miRNAs showing high expression levels in PCa tissues are reported as suitable diagnostic or prognostic markers [6]. Among deregulated miRNAs in PCa, some miRNAs are directly under androgen receptor (AR) signaling control and function as the effectors of androgen signaling [6]. Recent findings have shown apoptosis antagonizing transcription factor (AATF) gene encodes a miRNA designated as miR-2909 that plays an important role in immunity and cancer progression [7, 8]. AATF is known as co-activator of AR through its interaction via LXXLL motifs and therefore enhances the AR mediated transcription. AR signaling has a critical role in the development of normal prostate by triggering various events that promote epithelial cell growth, arrest and differentiation [9]. However, this pathway is modified/deregulated to promote cell survival and proliferation in PCa [10]. Keeping in view the critical role played by AR signaling in normal prostate and PCa development, human AATF genome, that holds AATF gene and its encoded miR-2909 within its fold, assumes huge importance. Exploring its role in PCa, miR-2909 was identified as an androgen-regulated miRNA acting as a novel mediator of androgen/androgen receptor signaling and exerting its oncogenic effects through multiple pathways. This chapter addresses the role played by miR-2909 in the progression of PCa and the potential signaling pathways through which it operates. The purpose of this chapter is mainly to bring into limelight the role played by one of the less known miRNAs to the readers which when combined with another set of miRNAs or specifically AR-regulated miRNAs could be exploited for therapeutic and diagnostic purposes, though further studies are demanded to obtain more definite conclusions.

2. Prostate gland structure and PCa types

Prostate is a compound tubuloalveolar exocrine gland that plays a vital role in the reproductive process by secreting a part of the seminal fluid. The average size of the prostate is about a size of a large walnut that is located close to the rectum, below the bladder at the base of the penis. The prostatic epithelium is composed of two major cell types: stromal cells and epithelial cells.

There are five types of cells present in prostate epithelium including stem cells, basal epithelial cells, transit-amplifying cells, neuroendocrine cells and secretory epithelial cells.

The stromal compartment, which normally serves as structural support, mainly consists of connective tissue, smooth muscle cells and fibroblasts. The gland can be divided into three glandular zones: the transition zone (TZ), the central zone (CZ) and the peripheral zone (PZ). The TZ consists of two lobes, accounting for 5% prostatic volume, whereas CZ is located outside the TZ and accounts for about 25% prostatic volume. Outside the CZ is the PZ which constitutes about 70% of the total prostatic volume. Most of the benign hyperplasias and 10–20% tumors arise in TZ whereas 70–75% of the prostate tumors arise in PZ. Acinar prostate carcinoma is the most common histological form whereas other subtypes only account for 5–10% of histological forms and include ductal adenocarcinoma, atrophic carcinoma, pseudo-hyperplastic carcinoma, foamy gland carcinoma, mucinous carcinoma, signet-ring carcinoma, small cell carcinoma, sarcomatoid carcinoma, urothelial carcinoma and squamous cell carcinoma.

3. MiRNAs

miRNAs are naturally occurring 18–24 nucleotides-long non-coding RNA molecules that regulate the expression of a large number of genes posttranscriptionally either through mRNA degradation or inhibition of translation [11]. miRNAs play an important role in a wide range of biological processes including cell proliferation, differentiation, development and apoptosis [12]. To date, approximately 2000 human miRNAs have been discovered and believed to regulate about 30% of human genes. miRNAs are known to regulate genes through three different mechanisms including triggering an endonucleolytic cleavage of mRNA, promoting translational repression or through accelerating the deadenylation of mRNA [11]. The endonucleolytic cleavage of target mRNAs is usually possible if the miRNA sequence is completely complementary to the target mRNA sequence although some mismatches could occur. However, translational repression occurs if there is a non-perfect match between the two sequences. Nucleotides 2–7 from the 5' end of the miRNA, called seed sequence, are essential to the binding of the miRNA to the target mRNA perfectly and all the other nucleotides of the miRNA can bind imperfectly. Though majority of data has focused on miRNAs that act via canonical pathway, there are no mechanistic requirements that restrict miRNA action to only 3'untranslated region (UTR). miRNAs have also been reported to regulate mRNA expression by targeting 5'UTR and open reading frame (ORF) binding sites. Moreover, various studies have reported miRNAs that directly bind to DNA and influence gene expression and some miRNAs are reported to even activate, rather than inhibit gene expression [13]. Altogether, these findings highlight the complexity of gene regulation by the miRNAs.

Lot of miRNAs are located in distinct regions far from protein-coding genes and expressed independently from their own promoters. However, 40% of miRNAs are located in introns of protein-coding genes and are under the control of same promoter and co-expressed with the host gene. Likewise, various miRNAs are located close to each other within 10 kb in the form of clusters. miRNAs are normally transcribed as monocistronic by polymerase II whereas clustered miRNAs are transcribed as polycistronic RNAs. The transcribed sequences are a few hundred to a few thousand nucleotides in length and are termed as preliminary miRNAs (pri-miRNAs). Pri-miRNAs harbor a polyadenyl-tail and have a 5′7-methylguanylate cap (95) at the 5′ end. The pri-miRNA synthesized is cleaved by the nuclear microprocessor complex formed by Drosha, a member of the RNase III family of enzymes, and the DiGeorge 21 critical region 8 proteins. If the seed sequence of miRNA and its target mRNA are highly complementary, mRNA degradation is induced via the RNAse III catalytic domain of the AGO proteins, which is followed by the degradation by exonuclease XRN1, the exosome and SKI complex. If the miRNA and mRNA are partially complementary, mRNA degradation is followed through different pathways. The poly(A) tail of the mRNA is deadenylated followed by degradation of the mRNA from the 3′ end by the cytoplasmic exonucleases degradation mechanism or by removal of 5′cap via decapping complex proteins (DCP1 and DCP2) and CAF1-CCR4-NOT complexes and then degradation of the mRNA by XRN1 from 5′ to 3′ end [11].

4. MiRNAs in PCa

As miRNAs have been associated with various important physiological processes like development, differentiation, apoptosis and cell cycle regulation, thus aberrant miRNA expression can result in various pathological states, including cancer [14]. Various studies have shown that different miRNAs and their targets are aberrantly expressed in neoplastic PCa tissues compared to the normal ones, providing a significant insight into altered cellular growth, invasion and metastatic potential of PCa cells [6, 15]. These miRNAs appear to have important and unique roles with respect to apoptosis resistance, cell proliferation, epithelial-to-mesenchymal transition, invasion, metastasis and development of androgen independence. These differentially expressed miRNAs function as either oncogenes or tumor suppressor genes with oncogenic being upregulated and tumor suppressors being downregulated. Various miRNA expression profiling analytical studies have shown many miRNAs downregulated in PCa wherein their elevated levels are indicators of good prognosis [6, 15]. On the contrary, other miRNAs are promoters of carcinogenesis and their expression levels are elevated in advanced stages of some cancers, which clearly suggests these miRNAs as attractive targets for therapy [6, 15]. Although a good number of miRNAs are reported as being differentially expressed in PCa, which in turn leads to altered expression and activity of their targets, the understanding of the functional importance of only several miRNAs has been molecularly exploited. Such studies have established an intimate relationship between PCa and miRNAs with emerging data clearly suggesting miRNAs a very promising field in terms of therapeutics, although further in-depth mechanistic studies and a better understanding of the key events are desired.

5. miR-2909

miR-2909, previously known as Che-1 and encoded by AATF gene, is known to regulate crucial genes involved in host immunity, energy metabolism and oncogenic/oncostatic activities

[8, 16]. AATF/Che-1 genome has emerged like a master epigenetic switch shown to regulate cell cycle progression, checkpoint control and apoptosis [17]. A new dimension was added to AATF Genome by a finding that AATF acts as co-activator of AR through its interaction via LXXLL motifs and thus enhances the AR mediated transcription. AR signaling has a critical role in the development of normal prostate by triggering various events that promote epithelial cell growth, arrest and differentiation [9]. However, this pathway is modified/deregulated to promote cell survival and proliferation in PCa [10]. Keeping in view the critical role played by AR signaling in normal prostate and PCa development, human AATF genome, holding AATF gene and its encoded miR-2909 within its fold, assumes huge importance. Further, various studies focused to explore the role of miR-2909 in PCa were conducted and the potential signaling pathways through which miR-2909 operates were explored. A new dimensional role was added to miR-2909 by various studies that revealed miR-2909 as an androgen-regulated miRNA acting as a novel mediator of androgen/androgen receptor (AR) signaling. miR-2909 enhanced the proliferation potential of PCa cells and assisted in PCa survival under reduced androgen levels by maintaining a positive feedback loop with AR. Further, miR-2909 was shown to exert it oncogenic effects by attenuating the tumor-suppressive effects of transforming growth factor beta (TGFβ) signaling by directly targeting transforming growth factor beta receptor 2 (TGFBR2) and via signal transducer and activator of transcription 1 (STAT1) pathway and by upregulating ISGylation pathway through SOCS3/STAT1 pathway.

6. miR-2909 and AR signaling

AR signaling plays a critical role in the development of normal prostate [9]. However, this pathway is deregulated to promote cancer development and progression in PCa patients. miR-2909 is identified as an androgen-induced miRNA that functions as a novel mediator of androgen/androgen receptor signaling. Comparison of AR negative, PC3 and AR positive LNCaP PCa cell lines has shown a three-fold higher expression of miR-2909 in LNCaP cell line. Further, androgens were observed to induce an enhanced expression of miR-2909 and androgen-deprivation downregulated miR-2909 expression in androgen-dependent LNCaP cells. Moreover, the expression level of miR-2909 also increased proportionately when LNCaP cells were treated with different concentrations of DHT ranging from 0.1–15 nM. Moreover, this androgen-mediated regulation of miR-2909 was executed through AR signaling. To rule out any cross-activation of Estrogen receptor-b (ERb) signaling, it was further shown that DHT induced miR-2909 expression was significantly blocked in the presence of AR antagonists, strongly indicating the involvement of AR in androgen-mediated regulation of miR-2909 expression. It was further suggested that a positive feedback loop operates between AR and miR-2909 in prostate cells (**Figure 1**). Ectopic expression of miR-2909 in AR-positive LNCaP cells resulted in significant upregulation and inhibition of endogenous miR-2909 significantly reduced the AR and PSA expression. It is a well-established fact that the expression of AR increases in prostate tumor cells. It could therefore be speculated that the positive feedback loop between AR and miR-2909 in prostate tumors could help to maintain a steady level of AR in the absence of androgens for further progression and development.

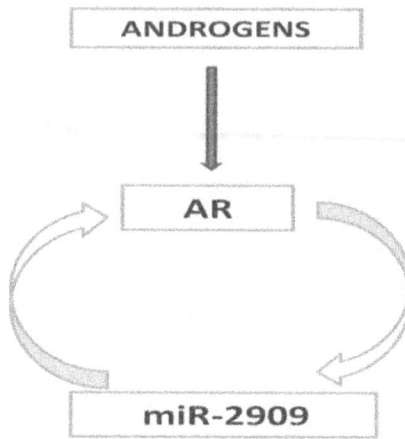

Figure 1. Feedback loop between androgen receptor and miR-2909.

7. miR-2909 stimulates androgen-dependent and androgen-independent growth

The functional analysis of miR-2909 in PCa was studied by transfecting miR-2909 into different PCa cell lines. Ectopic expression of miR-2909 enhanced the proliferation potential of both LNCaP and PC3 cells. The treatment of miR-2909-transfected LNCaP cells with an anti-androgen, bicalutamide significantly inhibited the cell proliferation rate. PCa commonly progresses from an androgen-dependent (AD) to an androgen-independent (AI) stage. Evaluating the role of miR-2909 in AI conditions, it was observed that miR-2909 overexpression significantly stimulated the growth of AD-LNCaP cells cultured in androgen-deprived medium and rescued them from androgen-ablated growth arrest. Similarly, anti-miR-2909 significantly inhibited the growth of AD LNCaP cells. Moreover, overexpression of miR-2909 significantly stimulated the growth of AR negative PC3 cells also.

8. miR-2909 and TGF beta signaling

In PCa, multiple AR mediated growth-regulatory signaling pathways are disrupted, disturbing the equilibrium between proliferation and apoptosis and tipping the balance in favor of proliferation. TGFβ signaling represents one of the important pathways AR cross talks with [18, 19]. Although various studies have shown that AR signaling blocks the TGFβ-induced inhibitory effects, however, exact molecular mechanisms are not known yet [20, 21]. We have for the first time reported in our study that miR-2909 acts as one of the central mediators of this cross talk [22]. TGFBR2, a critical signaling effector of TGFβ signaling, was shown as a novel putative target of miR-2909. TGFBR2 expression was downregulated in miR-2909 overexpressing PC3 cells and upregulated in anti-miR-2909-treated LNCaP cells. Ectopically

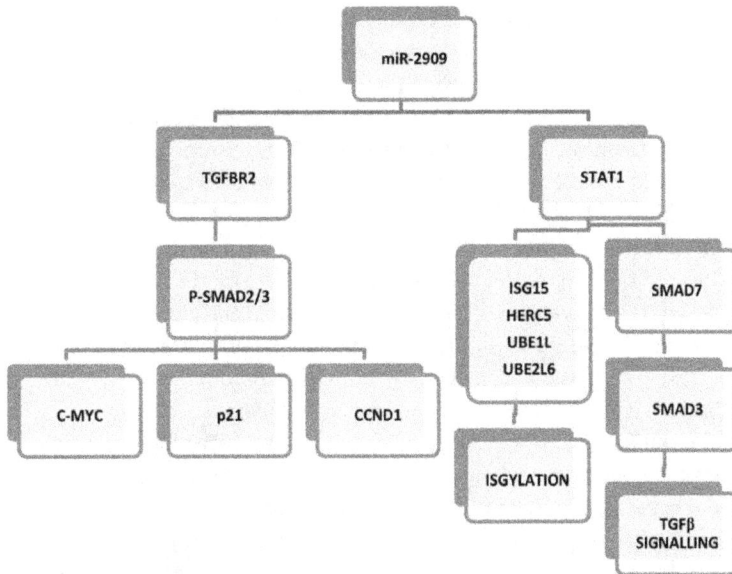

Figure 2. Schematic model summarizing the role of miR-2909 in PCa.

expressed miR-2909 decreased the basal phosphorylation of SMAD3, a downstream effector of TGFβ signaling and thus abrogating TGFβ-mediated cell growth inhibition and apoptosis in PC3 cells. Further, a significant upregulation of p21^{CIP} and downregulation of c-MYC and CCND1 expression was observed in TGFβ-treated PC3 cells and miR-2909 overexpression abrogated these TGFβ-mediated effects (**Figure 2**). Thus, these results suggest a novel mechanism of escaping tumor-suppressive effects of TGFβ signaling mediated through downregulation of TGFBR2 by miR-2909 alone or AR/miR-2909 axis which could be a vital mechanism for PCa cell survival and progression. Supporting this data, various studies have shown that downregulation of TGFBR2 induces malignant transformation while TGFBR2 activation promotes the pro-apoptotic function in vitro as well as in vivo [23, 24]. The significance of TGFβ pathway in castrate-resistant prostate cancer is further supported by various studies that have reported an association between reduced TGFBR2 expression with higher Gleason score and elevated risk of relapse or decreased survival rate after androgen depletion therapy in PCa patients [25, 26].

9. miR-2909 and ISGylation

ISG15 is an interferon-induced 165-amino-acid (17 kDa) protein that belongs to a ubiquitin-like protein superfamily [27]. Like ubiquitin, ISG15 has diverse functions including ISGylation, a ubiquitin-like modification process by which ISG15 covalently conjugates to cytoplasmic and nuclear proteins through its conserved LRLRGG sequence and alters their functional properties [28]. A significant upregulation of all components of ISGylation including ISG15,

HERC5, UBE1L and UBE2L6 were observed in miR-2909 over-expressing PC3 cells (**Figure 3**). Further, it was observed that miR-2909 overexpression modulated ISGylation through STAT1 mediated via negative regulation of SOCS3. A significant upregulation of STAT1 phosphorylation and downregulation of SOCS3 was detected in miR-2909-overexpressing PC3 cells whereas miR-2909 plasmid coupled with antagomiR-2909 treatment significantly downregulated phosphorylated STAT1 and upregulated SOCS3 expression [29]. The SOCS3 is a well-documented inhibitor of JAK/STAT pathway and STAT1 phosphorylation is always reported as inversely correlated with SOCS3 expression [30]. A pro-tumorigenic activity mediated by miR-2909-induced ISGylation upregulation via STAT1 is supported by various studies reporting constitutive STAT1 activation as tumor-promoting in multiple cancer models. A positive correlation between increasing STAT1 expression and pro-proliferative gene expression with increasing disease progression from benign human papilloma virus-negative and benign human papilloma virus-positive, malignant cervical squamous carcinoma cells have been reported [31]. A similar kind of correlation between STAT1 with increasing disease progression from ductal carcinoma in situ to invasive carcinoma in breast cancer biopsies has also been reported. Likewise, the STAT1 expression in human breast cancer has been reported to be a predictive marker of poor prognosis as well as chemotherapy and radiotherapy resistance [32, 33]. Ectopic expression of miR-2909 in PC3 cells increased their proliferation rate and silencing miR-2909-induced or endogenous level of ISGylation process in PCa cells significantly reduced the cell proliferation rate. Cell cycle analysis also revealed a significant decrease in fraction of cells in S phase, clearly indicating the effect of miR-2909 on cell proliferation could be partly mediated via ISGylation.

In support of these results, interferons have been shown to upregulate AR expression, a molecule known to play a critical role in PCa development and progression. Similarly, Kiessling et al. [34] have shown that UBE1L overexpression, one of the limiting components of ISGylation

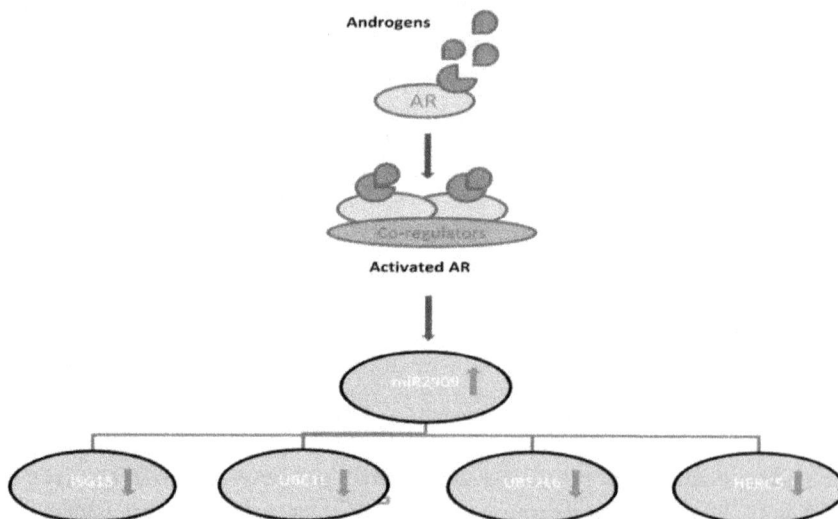

Figure 3. Downregulation of ISGylation through AR/miR-2909 axis in AR-positive LNCaP cells.

in LNCaP cells, increased AR levels in an ISG15-dependent manner. In breast cancer also, ISG15 is reported to stabilize oncogenic K-Ras protein via modifying it through ISGylation by inhibiting its targeted degradation via lysosomes [35]. All these observations clearly implicate that miR-2909 may very well play an important role in PCa progression through modulating ISGylation process.

Moreover, it is well-known that the signaling events triggered by TGF-β are negatively regulated by STAT1 through SMAD7 [36]. Phosphorylation of STAT1 induces transcription of SMAD7, which is a negative regulator for the cascade of SMAD3-mediated TGF-β signaling. miR-2909 overexpression significantly upregulated the expression of SMAD7 and decreased SMAD3 phosphorylation in PC3 cells (**Figure 2**). Moreover, the effect was reversed and the expression of SMAD3 resumed to normal levels when SMAD7 was inhibited using si-SMAD7. TGFβ is known to be a negative growth regulator that plays a critical role in PCa by controlling cell proliferation and apoptosis. An expanding body of evidence has indicated dysfunctional TGFβ signaling in various malignancies including PCa. Henceforth, all these studies suggest modulation of TGF-beta signaling by miR-2909 through multiple mechanisms. As ISGylation is known to play a pro-tumorigenic role and is also associated with poor prognosis, thus miR-2909 could serve as a potential prognostic biomarker for cancer patients. Further, the negative regulation of TGFβ signaling signifies that miR-2909 plays a pro-tumorigenic role by manipulating multiple signaling pathways. However, these studies represent the preliminary attempt and need to be further extended to human clinical PCa samples where these in vitro studies could be validated and the potential role of miR-2909 as a therapeutic biomarker could be established.

10. Urinary-exosomal miR-2909 and PCa

Exosomes are small membrane-bound vesicles of 40–100 nm in diameter found in a broad range of biological fluids. They play a critical role in cross talk between tumors and the surrounding environment. Various molecules encapsulated in these vesicles circulating in various body fluids are proteins and nucleic acids including mRNA and miRNAs [37, 38]. Various studies have reported a change in the content of freely circulating exosomal miRNAs during tumorigenesis reflecting the situation in the tumor [38]. Samina et al. [39] studied the relative urinary exosomal recruitment levels of two miRNAs, that is, mir-2909 & miR-615-3p in human subjects suffering from either bladder cancer or PCa. Urinary exosomes, derived from human subjects suffering from PCa, were found to be enriched with miR-2909 compared to those derived from either healthy control subjects or benign prostatic hyperplasia (BPH) subjects or patients with urinary bladder cancer. In contrast, miR-615-3p was significantly recruited to urinary exosomes in subjects suffering from both bladder and PCa compared to those found in either healthy-control subjects or disease-control subjects suffering from BPH. Elucidating the correlation of urinary exosomal miRNAs with PCa severity, the extent of miR-2909 recruitment to the urinary exosomes showed significant correlation with the severity of PCa based on Gleason Score within different subgroups grouped into Hormone-sensitive or Hormone-insensitive or Hormone-naive groups [39]. Further, in this study, it was reported that the serum PSA levels did not correlate with the severity of PCa either in Hormone-sensitive or Hormone-insensitive subjects. Moreover, no significant relationship between severity of PCa and age was observed. From this study, it can be implied that urinary-exosomal miR-2909 cannot only help to differentiate bladder cancer from PCa but can also help to know the aggressiveness of PCa.

11. Clinical applications

Currently, PSA measurement is the only routinely performed test for the diagnosis of PCa. PSA is a coagulase protein secreted by prostate epithelial cells into semen. When the level of PSA goes above 4 ng/ml, the subject is asked to go for prostate biopsy for further evaluation. However, the PSA testing is non-specific as elevated PSA levels due to BPH, infection and/or chronic inflammation may sometimes lead to confounding results leading to over-diagnosis and over-treatment for insignificant tumors. Moreover, PSA measurement can also give false negative results as sometimes the patients suffering from PCa show a PSA level within normal range, thus leading to wrong diagnosis. Another important limitation of PSA testing is its lack of ability to identify aggressive and lethal forms of PCa. Thus, even though PSA is a valuable tool, it lacks specificity and is therefore not considered an optimal biomarker. Therefore, novel biomarkers are extremely desired due to the limitations of PSA.

The current research scenario gives compelling reasons to believe that miRNAs could serve as potential therapeutic tools in the form of monotherapy or in combination therapy with the available medical treatments. miRNAs alone or allied with PSA testing can serve together as potential biomarker for the accurate diagnosis of PCa [40, 41]. From the above studies, it can be implied that detection and quantification of miR-2909 alone or in combination with other miRNAs could serve as a reliable, non-invasive biofluid-based diagnostic test that can help to determine the presence and nature of a prostate malignancy as well as its response to treatment. However, it is to be insisted that a good number of investigational studies based on larger number of patients are needed to obtain more definite conclusions.

12. Conclusion

Collectively, miR-2909 is an androgen-inducible miRNA that forms a positive loop with AR and helps in prostate cancer progression. miR-2909 exerts its oncogenic effects via multiple mechanisms including attenuation of tumor-suppressive effects of TGFβ signaling and by upregulating ISGylation pathway. Moreover, it can be speculated that the recruitment of miR-2909 within the urinary exosomes in PCa patients can act as a non-invasive diagnostic marker for all the traits of PCa severity.

Author details

Shiekh Gazalla Ayub

Address all correspondence to: gazallakhan@ymail.com

Venus Remedies, Panchkula, India

References

[1] Worldwide Cancer Statistics. Cancer Research UK. 2015. Available from: http://www. cancerresearchuk.org/health-professional/cancer-statistics/worldwide-cancer [Accessed: October 19, 2017]

[2] Prostate Cancer Estimated Incidence, Mortality and Prevalence Worldwide in 2012. GLOBOCAN Cancer Fact Sheets: Prostate Cancer. Available from: http://globocan. iarc. fr/old/FactSheets/cancers/prostate-new.asp [Accessed: October 19, 2017]

[3] Yeole BB. Trends in the prostate cancer incidence in India. Asian Pacific Jornal of Cancer Prevention APJCP. 2008;**9**(1):141-144

[4] Hans L, David U, Vickers Andrew J. Prostate-specific antigen and prostate cancer: Prediction, detection and monitoring. Nature Reviews Cancer. 2008;**8**(4):268-278. DOI: 10.1038/ nrc2351

[5] Lucas N, Renato C, Eastham James A. Other biomarkers for detecting prostate cancer. BJU International. 2010;**105**(2):166-169. DOI: 10.1111/j.1464-410X.2009.09088.x

[6] Gazalla AS, Deepak K, Taha A. Microdissecting the role of microRNAs in the pathogenesis of prostate cancer. Cancer Genetics. 2015;**208**(6):289-302. DOI: 10.1016/j.cancergen. 2015.02.010

[7] Deepak K, Mansi A, Anuradha G, Sharma S. MALT1 induced immune response is governed by miR-2909 RNomics. Molecular Immunology. 2014:**64**. DOI: 10.1016/j.molimm. 2014.11.018

[8] Deepti M, Deepak K, Nalini C, Kumar MR. miR-2909-mediated regulation of KLF4: A novel molecular mechanism for differentiating between B-cell and T-cell pediatric acute lymphoblastic leukemias. Molecular Cancer. 2014;**13**:175. DOI: 10.1186/1476-4598-13-175

[9] Simeng W, Hong-Chiang C, Jing T, Zhiqun S, Yuanjie N, Chawnshang C. Stromal androgen receptor roles in the development of normal prostate, benign prostate hyperplasia, and prostate cancer. American Journal of Pathology. 2015;**185**(2):293-301. DOI: 10.1016/j. ajpath.2014.10.012

[10] Lonergan Peter E, Tindall DJ. Androgen receptor signaling in prostate cancer development and progression. Journal of Carcinogenesis. 2011;**10**:20. DOI: 10.4103/1477-3163.83937

[11] Stefanie J, Elisa I. Towards a molecular understanding of microRNA-mediated gene silencing. Nature Review Genetics. 2015;**16**(7):421-433. DOI: 10.1038/nrg3965

[12] Yimei C, Yu X, Hu S, Yu J. A brief review on the mechanisms of miRNA regulation. Genomics, Proteomics and Bioinformatics. 2009;**7**(4):147-154. DOI: 10.1016/S1672-0229 (08)60044-3

[13] Place Robert F, Long-Cheng L, Deepa P, Noonan Emily J, Rajvir D. MicroRNA-373 induces expression of genes with complementary promoter sequences. Proceedings of the National Academy of Sciences. 2008;**105**(5):1608-1613. DOI: 10.1073/pnas.0707594105

[14] Ardekani Ali M, Moslemi NM. The role of MicroRNAs in human diseases. Avicenna Journal of Medical Biotechnology. 2010;2(4):161-179

[15] Daniela V, Mariarosaria B, Sabrina R, Carla C, Carmine D'A, Rossella DF, et al. Micrornas in prostate cancer. An overview. Oncotarget. 2017;8(30):50240-50251. DOI. 10.10632/oncotarget.16933

[16] Deepak K, Sugandha S. High glucose-induced human cellular immune response is governed by miR-2909 RNomics. Blood Cells Molecules and Diseases. 2015;54(4):342-347. DOI: 10.1016/j.bcmd.2015.01.009

[17] Simona I, Maurizio F. Discovering Che-1/AATF: A new attractive target for cancer therapy. Frontiers in Genetics. 2015;6:141. DOI: 10.3389/fgene.2015.00141

[18] Zheng C, Natasha K. Mechanisms navigating the TGF-β pathway in prostate cancer. Asian Journal of Urology. 2015;2(1):11-18. DOI: 10.1016/j.ajur.2015.04.011

[19] Zhu M-L, Natasha K. Androgen receptor and growth factor signaling cross-talk in prostate cancer cells. Endocrine Related Cancer. 2008;15(4):841-849. DOI: 10.1677/ERC-08-0084

[20] Hayes SA, Zarnegar M, Sharma M, Yang F, Peehl DM, ten Dijke P, et al. SMAD3 represses androgen receptor-mediated transcription. Cancer Research. 2001;61(5):2112-2118

[21] Lucia MS, Sporn MB, Roberts AB, Stewart LV, Danielpour D. The role of transforming growth factor-beta1, -beta2, and -beta3 in androgen-responsive growth of NRP-152 rat prostatic epithelial cells. Journal of Cell Physiology. 1998;175(2):184-192. DOI: 10.1002/(SICI)1097-4652(199805)175:2<184::AID-JCP8>3.0.CO;2-K

[22] Gazalla AS, Deepak K, Taha A. An androgen-regulated miR-2909 modulates TGFβ signalling through AR/miR-2909 axis in prostate cancer. Gene. 2017;631:1-9. DOI: 10.1016/j.gene.2017.07.037

[23] Yang H, Zhang H, Zhong Y, Wang Q, Yang L, Kang H, et al. Concomitant underexpression of TGFBR2 and overexpression of hTERT are associated with poor prognosis in cervical cancer. Scientific Reports. 2017;7:e41670. DOI: 10.1038/srep41670

[24] Hong P, Joanne C, Elisabeth J, Dustin G, Shinichi S, Adam V, et al. Dysfunctional transforming growth factor-β receptor II accelerates prostate tumorigenesis in the TRAMP mouse model. Cancer Research. 2009;69(18):7366-7374. DOI: 10.1158/0008-5472.CAN-09-0758

[25] Teixeira Ana L, Mónica G, Augusto N, Azevedo Andreia S, Joana A, Francisca D, et al. Improvement of a predictive model of castration-resistant prostate cancer: Functional genetic variants in TGFβ1 signaling pathway modulation. PLoS One. 2013;8(8):e72419. DOI: 10.1371/journal.pone.0072419

[26] Guo Y, Jacobs Stephen C, Natasha K. Down-regulation of protein and mRNA expression for transforming growth factor-β (TGF-β1) type I and type II receptors in human prostate cancer. International Journal of Cancer. 1997;71(4):573-579. DOI: 10.1002/(SICI)1097-0215(19970516)71:4<573::AID-IJC11>3.0.CO;2-D

[27]   Korant BD, Blomstrom DC, Korant BD, Blomstrom DC, Jonak GJ, Knight E Jr. Interferon-induced proteins. Purification and characterization of a 15 000-dalton protein from human and bovine cells induced by interferon. Journal of Biological Chemistry. **259**:14835-14839

[28]   Chen Z, Carilee D, Huibregtse Jon M, Steven G, Krug Robert M. Human ISG15 conjugation targets both IFN-induced and constitutively expressed proteins functioning in diverse cellular pathways. Proceedings of the National Academy of Sciences of the United States of America. 2005;**102**(29):10200-10205. DOI: 10.1073/pnas.0504754102

[29]   Gazalla AS, Deepak K. miR-2909 regulates ISGylation system via STAT1 signalling through negative regulation of SOCS3 in prostate cancer. Andrology. 2017;**5**(4):790-797. DOI: 10.1111/andr.12374

[30]   The Suppressor of Cytokine Signaling (SOCS) 1 and SOCS3 but Not SOCS2 Proteins Inhibit Interferon-mediated Antiviral and Antiproliferative Activities. n.d. Available from: http://www.jbc.org/content/273/52/35056.long [Accessed: May 31, 2016]

[31]   Mahmood M, Gernot H, Anneliese F-R, Daphne G-K, Kerstin P, Klaus C. Gene profiling in pap-cell smears of high-risk human papillomavirus-positive squamous cervical carcinoma. Gynaecologic Oncology. 2007;**105**(2):418-426. DOI: 10.1016/j.ygyno.2006.12.032

[32]   Khodarev N, Ahmad R, Rajabi H, Pitroda S, Kufe T, McClary C, et al. Cooperativity of the MUC1 oncoprotein and STAT1 pathway in poor prognosis human breast cancer. Oncogene. 2010;**29**(6):920-929. DOI: 10.1038/onc.2009.391

[33]   Weichselbaum Ralph R, Hemant I, Taewon Y, Nuyten Dimitry SA, Baker Samuel W, Nikolai K, et al. An interferon-related gene signature for DNA damage resistance is a predictive marker for chemotherapy and radiation for breast cancer. Proceedings of the National Academy of Sciences of the United States of America. 2008;**105**(47):18490-18495. DOI: 10.1073/pnas.0809242105

[34]   Kiessling A, Hogrefe C, Erb S, Bobach C, Fuessel S, Wessjohann L, et al. Expression, regulation and function of the ISGylation system in prostate cancer. Oncogene. 2009;**28**(28):2606-2620. DOI: 10.1038/onc.2009.115

[35]   Burks J, Reed RE, Desai SD. ISGylation governs the oncogenic function of Ki-Ras in breast cancer. Oncogene. 2014;**33**(6):794-803. DOI: 10.1038/onc.2012.633

[36]   Seok-Rae P, Mee-Hyeun J, Seong-Hyun J, Mi-Hee P, Kyoung-Hoon P, Lee M-R, et al. IFN-gamma down-regulates TGF-beta1-induced IgA expression through Stat1 and p300 signaling. Molecules and Cells. 2010;**29**(1):57-62. DOI: 10.1007/s10059-010-0004-4

[37]   Kelly Brian D, Nicola M, Healy Nuala A, Kilian W, Kerin Michael J. A review of expression profiling of circulating microRNAs in men with prostate cancer. BJU International. 2013;**111**(1):17-21. DOI: 10.1111/j.1464-410X.2012.11244.x

[38]   Selth Luke A, Tilley Wayne D, Butler LM. Circulating microRNAs: Macro-utility as markers of prostate cancer? Endocrine Related Cancer. 2012;**19**(4):R99-R113. DOI: 10.1530/ERC-12-0010

[39] Wani S, Kaul D, Mavuduru RS, Kakkar N, Bhatia A. Urinary-exosomal miR-2909: A novel pathognomonic trait of prostate cancer severity. Journal of Biotechnology. 2017;**259**:135-139. DOI: 10.1016/j.jbiotec.2017.07.029

[40] Lodes Michael J, Marcelo C, Dominic S, Sandra M, Amit K, Brooke A. Detection of cancer with serum miRNAs on an oligonucleotide microarray. PLoS One. 2009;**4**(7):e6229. DOI: 10.1371/journal.pone.0006229

[41] Brase Jan C, Marc J, Thorsten S, Maria F, Alexander H, Thomas S, et al. Circulating miRNAs are correlated with tumor progression in prostate cancer. International Journal of Cancer. 2011;**128**(3):608-616. DOI: 10.1002/ijc.25376

Chapter 5

Development of Oncolytic Adenoviruses for the Management of Prostate Cancer

Ahmed A. Ali and Gunnel Halldén

Additional information is available at the end of the chapter

http://dx.doi.org/10.5772/intechopen.73515

Abstract

Prostate cancer (PCa) is the fifth most common cause of cancer-related deaths in men globally. Androgen receptor (AR) signalling plays a vital role in initiation and progression and antiandrogens are standard of care first-line therapeutics. However, resistance frequently develops resulting in metastatic castration-resistant prostate cancer (mCRPC). Management of CRPC is currently chemotherapy and/or radiotherapy but is mostly palliative due to rapid development of resistance. The need for novel approaches to eliminate mCRPC is compelling; a promising option is replication-selective (oncolytic) adenoviruses with demonstrated efficacy in preclinical models of multidrug-resistant PCa. The safety of various viral mutants has been confirmed in numerous clinical trials with minimal toxicity in patients. Importantly, oncolytic adenoviruses synergise with the current standard of care for mCRPC even in treatment-resistant cells. In early phase I–II clinical trials, promising efficacy in patients with localised PCa was reported after intratumoural administration, and phase III trials are underway. To enable systemic delivery, for targeting of mCRPC, further developments are necessary because of the short half-life of the adenoviral mutants in human blood. Current progress in preventing the high-affinity binding of adenovirus to erythrocytes, hepatocyte uptake, and elimination by hepatic Kupffer cells will be described.

Keywords: prostate cancer, oncolytic adenoviruses, androgen, treatment resistance, viral modifications

1. Introduction

The current treatment approaches for prostate cancer (PCa) are successfully managing local disease with a reported 5-year survival rate of 100% [1]. At this stage, the treatment options are surgery (radical prostatectomy), radiation therapy, and androgen deprivation therapy (ADT), which includes castration, androgen receptor (AR) inhibition, and combined therapies. Castration is classified as either surgical (orchiectomy) or medical, for example, administration of luteinizing hormone-releasing hormone (LHRH) agonists or antagonists. Current use of AR inhibitors includes the nonsteroidal antiandrogens (NSAA) nilutamide, flutamide, and bicalutamide, which have demonstrated better tolerability than earlier steroidal antiandrogens such as cyproterone acetate. Combined androgen blockade (CAB) refers to the use of castration and AR antagonists combined [2]. In contrast, late-stage hormone-independent metastatic PCa has a 5-year survival rate of only 29% because of the development of resistance to all current therapeutics including cytotoxic drugs [1]. There is an unmet medical need for management of late-stage PCa. Efforts to improve the survival of patients with metastatic PCa have led to the development of novel therapeutics with the majority of agents targeting the androgen pathway, for example, the NSAA ARN-509 (Aragon Pharmaceuticals) and the androgen synthesis inhibitor abiraterone [3, 4]. However, only limited survival benefits and development of resistance have been observed with the new agents. A promising novel class of therapeutics that act through entirely different mechanisms than traditional cytotoxic and targeted drugs is oncolytic viruses. Currently, no oncolytic virus has been approved for treatment of PCa, although numerous phase I–II trials have been completed with promising outcomes and phase III trials are underway [5]. The most promising preclinical and clinical efficacy has been reported for various PCa-selective replicating adenoviral mutants that lyse cancer cells and leave normal cells unharmed and, in addition, resensitise drug-resistant cancer cells to chemotherapeutics [6–8].

1.1. Oncolytic viruses and prostate cancer

Gene therapy with oncolytic viruses is currently one of the most promising approaches for cancer elimination based on both preclinical data and results from numerous clinical trials. While classical gene therapy uses nonreplicating viruses as vectors to deliver transgenes to cancer cells, oncolytic virus therapy employs the lytic properties of replicating viruses to lyse cancer cells in addition to expression of cytotoxic transgenes to enhance efficacy and spread within the tumours [9]. Oncolytic viruses are engineered to replicate selectively in tumour cells and are most often genetically modified to selectively infect, propagate, and kill cancer cells without affecting normal cells [9, 10].

The concept of using replicating viruses in cancer treatment is not new; over a century ago, it was noted that tumours regressed in patients after naturally occurring systemic viral infections [10, 11]. During 1950–1980, several clinical trials were carried out to assess the ability of wild-type viruses to eliminate cancer, including the yellow fever, hepatitis, adenoviruses, and West Nile fever viruses [12]. However, the outcomes were not conclusive due to failure of infection control and spread to both healthy and malignant cells with poor patient outcomes. At present, it is well known that most cancer cells have impaired innate immune responses with decreased protection for viral infection, for example, altered interferon activity, resulting in enhanced viral replication in cancer cells compared to normal cells [13]. For this reason, the main challenges with viral therapies today are to prevent replication in normal cells rather than increase replication in tumour cells (**Figure 1**).

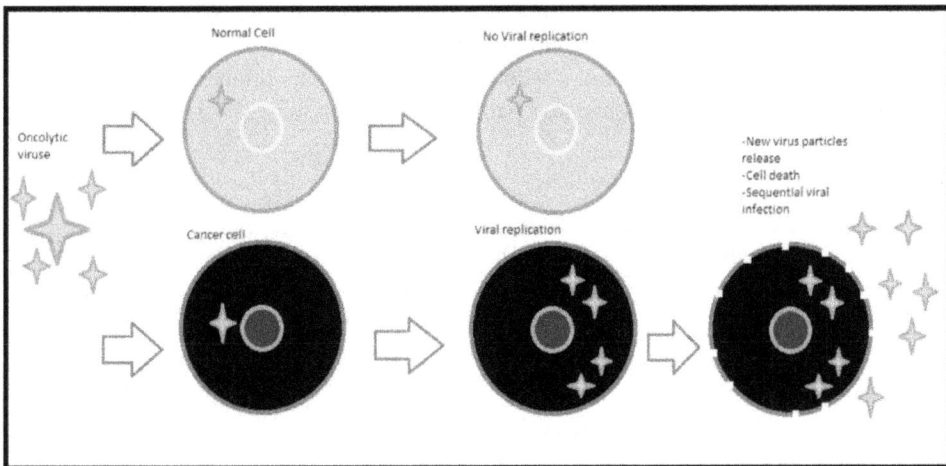

Figure 1. Selective replication and killing of cancer cells. Oncolytic viruses are engineered to replicate only in cancer cells by deleting viral genes that are essential for viral propagation in normal cells and are complemented in cancer cells by the altered gene expression in tumours. Alternatively, tumour-specific promoters are inserted in the viral genome to drive viral gene expression and propagation in cancer cells only. While oncolytic viruses may infect normal healthy cells viral propagation cannot proceed. In contrast, in cancer cells, viral infection leads to potent viral gene expression, genome amplification and virion assembly followed by virus-induced cell lysis and spread to surrounding tumour tissue.

In order to generate viruses that are cancer-selective, the functions of the viral gene-products must be fully understood to enable selection of the appropriate genes for engineering. One of the first oncolytic viral mutants for targeting of cancer cells was generated in 1991, by Martuza et al. [14]. The virus, a herpes simplex virus type 1 (HSVI) deleted in the thymidine kinase (TK) gene, which is essential for replication in normal cells, demonstrated good results in killing human glioblastoma cells both *in vitro* and in models *in vivo* [14]. A modified adenovirus, Oncorine or H101 (based on Onyx-015; [15]), was the first genetically engineered oncolytic virus to be approved for cancer therapy [16]. In 2005, the Chinese FDA granted market approval for Oncorine as an anticancer agent for hepatic and head and neck cancers. The phase III clinical trial that led to the approval assessed the benefits of adding Oncorine to cisplatin-based chemotherapy in the treatment of advanced head and neck squamous cell tumours by intratumoural administration. The objective response rates for the combination treated group were reported at 79%, while cisplatin alone resulted in 40% regression of injected tumours. However, no overall survival benefits were observed. The only other oncolytic virus on the market is Imlygic or T-VEC (Amgen), an HSVI mutant expressing granulocyte-macrophage colony-stimulating factor (GM-CSF) [17]. Imlygic was licenced in 2015 for melanoma by the FDA and approved in Europe in 2016 and in Australia in 2015. Currently, there are several engineered oncolytic viruses undergoing phase III clinical trials including a poxvirus (Pexa-Vec; JX-594; Transgene) for advanced hepatocellular carcinoma and the adenovirus mutant (CG0070; Cold Genesys) for bladder cancer [10]. During 2001–2014, six clinical trials investigating oncolytic virus therapy for recurrent localised prostate cancer were reported; four of them evaluated adenovirus-based therapies and two reovirus-based therapies, summarised in **Table 1** [18–23].

Currently, several phase I–II trials are ongoing using modified oncolytic adenoviruses. Although the development and use of oncolytic viruses have resulted in promising preclinical and clinical results, several challenges remain such as premature elimination of virus by the host immune system, viral pathogenic mechanisms, and failure to target all lesions at metastatic sites.

Virus	Genetic modifications	Phase/number of patients	Toxicity/route of administration	Outcomes
CV706	E1A expression controlled by PSA-promoter-enhancer	Phase I 20	Low Intraprostatic	65% of the patients had >30% serum PSA reduction and 25% had >50% serum PSA reduction [18]
CG7870	E1A expression controlled by rat-probasin-promoter E1B expression controlled by PSA-promoter-enhancer	Phase I 23	Grade 1 or 2, 13% grade 3 Intravenous	27% without PSA progression at 6 months, median time to PSA progression 60 days [19]
Ad5-CD/TK*rep*	E1B55K-deleted, armed with suicide genes (herpes simplex type 1 thymidine kinase cytosine deaminase)	Phase I 16	Grade 1 or 2 Intraprostatic	44% had ≥25% decrease in serum PSA level; 19% had ≥50% decrease in serum PSA level [20]
Ad5-CD/TK*rep*	E1B55K-deleted, armed with suicide genes (herpes simplex type 1 thymidine kinase cytosine deaminase)	Phase II 44	Grade 1 or 2 Intraprostatic	≥2 years after treatment, reduced biopsy positivity overall from actual biopsies (42%) and intention-to-treat (34%), and men with <50% biopsy positivity 60% [21]
Ad5-yCD/mutTK(SR39)rep-hNIS	E1B55K-deleted, hNIS as a reporter gene to monitor virus replication and efficacy	Phase I	Ongoing	Ongoing [59]
Ad5-yCD/mutTK(SR39)rep-hIL12	E1B-55K-deleted, armed with IL12	Phase I	Ongoing	Ongoing [60]
Reolysin®	None (wild type)	Phase I 5	Grade 1 and 2 Intravenous	51% decrease in PSA level in one patient with prostate cancer [22]
Reolysin®	None (wild type)	Phase I 4	Low, dose-limiting grade 4 neutropenia in one patient Intravenous	30% decrease in PSA level [23]

Table 1. Published prostate cancer clinical trials with oncolytic viruses.

2. Development of oncolytic adenoviruses

The most promising oncolytic viruses are genetically modified adenoviruses. Adenoviral mutants are continuously being developed to further improve on selectivity and efficacy. Adenovirus was discovered in the 1950s when it was isolated from adenoid tissues [24]. The linear double-stranded DNA genome, 30–38 kb, is enclosed in a protein capsid, forming 70–100 nm virion particles with icosahedral symmetry. There are more than 50 subtypes of the human adenovirus family that infect a broad range of host tissues often causing acute mild disease including respiratory infections, epidemic conjunctivitis, and infantile gastroenteritis [25, 26]. Despite the ability of certain subtypes to induce cancer in rodent models and transform cultured cells, there is no evidence to date that adenoviruses cause cancer in humans [27]. Currently, most clinical and preclinical studies have employed adenoviral mutants generated from type 5 (Ad5) because of its proven safety record and known functions.

2.1. Structure of adenoviruses

The viral capsid consists of 240 hexon and 12 penton proteins with fibre proteins projecting from the pentons and several small proteins that aid in stabilising the icosahedral structure [28]. The DNA containing core harbours additional proteins, the major polypeptide V and VII, a minor arginine-rich protein μ, which is covalently attached to the 5′-ends of the DNA, and the terminal proteins that bind to the DNA ends to act as primers for DNA replication. The viral DNA is wrapped around polypeptide VII similar to human DNA and histone proteins, and polypeptide V binds to the pentons to serve as a bridge between the core and the capsid.

The first adenoviral genome to be sequenced was from subtype 2 (Ad2), composed of 35,937 base pairs (bp) [29]. Since then, the majority of subtypes have been sequenced and found to have similar genome organisation and functional gene products as Ad2, including Ad5. The genome is divided into early expressed units (E1A, E1B, E2A, E2B, E3, and E4), delayed early units (IX and IVa2), and late units (L1–L5). The early units are the first to be expressed and encode proteins responsible for initiating transcription of other viral genes and for changing the intracellular environment to support viral production [30, 31]. The E1A proteins are required for productive infection and induce S-phase, cellular DNA synthesis and activate viral gene expression. The E2 proteins code for the viral DNA polymerase, which is essential for viral genome amplification. The E3 and E4 proteins are not essential for viral replication but prevent premature cell death of infected cells in response to the host immune defence and inhibit the DNA-damage repair, respectively. The late regions encode the viral structural proteins after viral genome amplification to encapsulate newly synthesised viral DNA. The VA RNA I and II reduce stimulation of the interferon response, delay cellular microRNA processing, and control the expression of host genes. Both ends of the genome contain the 100 bp inverted terminal repeats (ITRs), which serve as the origin of replication, and the viral packaging sequence (~200 bp), which is located next to the left ITR.

The viral particle enters the host cell through receptor-mediated endocytosis due to the interactions between the viral fibre and coxsackievirus and adenovirus receptor (CAR), and between pentons and integrins, mainly $\alpha v\beta 3$ and $\alpha v\beta 5$. The viral DNA is released in the endosome and transported to the nucleus where E1A is expressed constitutively, initiating expression of other early genes and hijacking the host cell DNA-synthesis machinery [31]. After complete viral genome amplification and assembly of new particles, the host cell is lysed and viruses spread and infect surrounding cells [32].

2.2. Anticancer activity of adenoviruses

Clinical evaluation of adenoviruses as oncolytic therapeutics started shortly after the discovery in the 1950s [11, 33]. The small genome is easy to engineer with known functions of the majority of the gene products, the genome is not integrated into the host cell DNA, the clinical safety profile is excellent with only flu-like side effects, and the natural tropism to epithelial cells renders adenocarcinomas, including PCa, excellent targets. Clinical developments have been limited to some extent because of the frequent downregulation of the native adenovirus receptor CAR in many tumours and the presence of preexisting antiadenoviral antibodies. A majority of the population has been infected with adenovirus at some point [27]. Several approaches have been explored to solve these limitations and are described below.

2.2.1. Viral fibre modifications

A promising and now common strategy that has been assessed in both preclinical and clinical studies is the modification of various regions of the viral capsid to enhance the affinity and therapeutic effects in CAR-negative cancer cell lines [27]. Several teams have evaluated fibre modifications that incorporate a partial peptide sequence from fibronectin, containing an arginine-glycine-aspartate-4C (RGD-4C) motif into the HI-loop of the fibre-knob, which enhances binding to $\alpha v\beta 3$- and $\alpha v\beta 5$-integrins and enables CAR-independent uptake [34]. RGD-modified viruses have improved oncolytic actions compared to unmodified virus in CAR-negative cancer cells. This strategy has proven to be efficacious for targeting of several solid cancers [35].

2.2.2. Chimeric viruses

The strategy of generating chimeric mutants has the advantage of employing multiple binding motifs from various parental viruses resulting in a broader transduction range of host cells [36]. For example, ovarian cancer cells were more efficiently targeted by adenovirus type 3 (Ad3) that binds to receptors including CD46 and CD80/CD86, but not CAR, and the Ad3 fibre was subsequently inserted in Ad5 to replace the native Ad5 fibre [36, 37]. The resulting chimeric Ad5/3 was more efficient in targeting ovarian cancer cells than Ad5 [38].

2.2.3. Antibody fusion constructs

A novel approach to improve adenovirus selectivity is the use of antibody fusion constructs, where two antibodies are used; one targets adenovirus capsid proteins, for example, using an antifibre knob antibody, and the other targets specific membrane receptors on the tumour cells [32, 33]. One promising cellular target antigen is the folate receptor, which is overexpressed in breast, ovarian, lung, and brain cancer cells [39]. This strategy resulted in improved selectivity and higher affinity of adenovirus to the tumour cells. A disadvantage of this technique is that the antibody binding to virus is lost in the progeny virions.

2.2.4. Complementation deletions

The most common strategy to generate replication-selective oncolytic adenoviral mutants is by introducing mutations in viral genes that are vital for replication in normal cells but are complemented by the altered cell cycle regulation in tumour cells (**Figure 1**). The first oncolytic adenovirus that was generated (*dl*1520, Onyx-015) was constructed by deleting the viral E1B55K protein, which binds to cellular p53 [15]. Inactivation of p53 is vital for adenovirus replication in normal cells to prevent apoptosis as a defence response to viral infection. In most cancers, p53 is nonfunctional through either direct mutations or mutations of p53-regulatory proteins [40]. It was demonstrated that adenoviral mutants that do not express E1B55K replicate exclusively in cancer cells lacking functional p53. Several versions of E1B55K-deleted mutants have shown promising oncolytic activity in spite of attenuated viral replication in numerous solid cancers. It is now known that E1B55K is crucial for the export of viral mRNA from the nucleus, giving a rational explanation for the limited replication of the virus in cancer cells [41]. Ongoing work is aimed at designing mutants with nonattenuating deletions to improve replication and efficacy in cancer cells. An example is the E1ACR2-deleted mutants that replicate selectively in cells with deregulated pRb-p16 pathway [42, 43]. The deletion of the small pRb-binding CR2-region in the E1A gene prevents binding to pRb, and thus these mutants cannot replicate in normal cells. Several versions of oncolytic adenovirus based on the deletion of E1ACR2 (e.g., Ad5/3Δ24hCG) have been designed and are under clinical evaluation for different types of cancers [43].

3. Prostate cancer–specific oncolytic adenoviruses

Oncolytic adenoviruses provide a promising treatment option for PCa due to their unique mode of action that synergises with current treatment modalities. There are two successful approaches that have been explored when targeting PCa. The first approach was to drive viral replication by prostate-specific promoters replacing the native viral promoter; this strategy is feasible because of the frequent overexpression of AR-regulated genes such as the prostate-specific antigen (PSA) and prostate-specific membrane antigen (PSMA) [44, 45]. Numerous viruses have been developed utilising various combinations of androgen-response elements (ARE) present in these genes [46]. The second strategy is the complementation deletions (see Section 2.2.4).

3.1. Prostate-specific antigen (PSA) regulatory elements

Several specific PSA regulatory elements have been explored to control adenovirus replication, including AREs and the PSA enhancer, which are located upstream of the promoter. The mutant CG7060 was constructed to express E1A from the PSA promoter/enhancer and showed selective replication and cell killing in prostate cancer cells [44]. In animal models using the PCa cell line LNCaP (AR-positive, PSA-expressing), tumour xenografts were grown in mice and were injected intratumourally with CG7060. During the first 2 weeks, the tumour volume increased slightly followed by a rapid decrease in growth. By 6 weeks, 50% of the mice were tumour-free [44]. In a clinical trial including 20 patients with locally recurrent PCa, CG7060 showed an acceptable safety profile and was not associated with significant toxicity (<grade 3) [18]. In addition, promising anticancer activity was suggested based on the reduction in PSA levels. A more recent and improved version of the CG7060 virus is CG7870, which has the PSA enhancer/promoter controlling E1B expression, while E1A expression is regulated by the rat probasin promoter (AR-regulated) [47]. CG7870 replicates 10^4–10^5 times more efficiently in PSA-positive cells than in PSA-negative cells, which is translated into 10,000 times higher cell killing activity [7, 48]. CG7870 was assessed in phase I and II trials for the management of locally recurrent prostate cancer through intratumoural administration and in hormone refractory metastatic prostate cancer through intravenous administration [19, 49]. In both settings, CG7870 was reported to significantly reduce PSA levels. Moreover, CG7870 synergised with other DNA-damaging therapies including radiotherapy or taxane chemotherapy in preclinical models [5, 7, 48].

3.2. Prostate-specific membrane antigen (PSMA) regulatory elements

PSMA is expressed in the prostate epithelial cell membrane and is significantly elevated in PCa cells compared to normal prostate cells and parallels the increases in Gleason score [50]. There are two identified transcriptional regulatory elements: the PSMA enhancer core (PSME) in the third intron of the PSMA gene (FOLH1) and the 1.2 kb upstream promoter of FOLH1 [51]. PSME is the key element for the prostate-specific expression of PSMA and is negatively regulated by androgens, which explains the high level of PSMA in prostate cancer after castration, unlike the PSA enhancers/promoters, which depend on androgen for activity [52]. The feasibility of using PSME as a regulatory element to control viral replication in PCa tissue has been evaluated by constructing the mutant Ad5-PSME-E1A with replication regulated by PSME-driven expression of E1A [52]. Castrated mice with prostate tumour xenografts received an intratumoural injection of Ad5-PSME-E1A or control virus, resulting in significant tumour regression only in Ad5-PSME-E1A-treated animals [52]. These outcomes suggest that PSME-mediated oncolytic adenovirus may be a promising strategy for management of PCa patients after hormonal therapy failure.

3.3. Prostate-specific chimeric regulatory elements

To further improve on the selectivity of viral mutants, chimeric prostate-specific enhancer-promoter elements were generated and explored [44, 53]. The combination of regulatory elements from PSA and PSMA was named prostate-specific enhancing sequence (PSES) and was inserted in Ad5 to generate Ad-UI1 and Ad-UI2 with the E1A and E4 genes controlled by the PSES [53]. Ad-UI1 is armed with the prodrug-converting enzyme thymidine kinase (TK) from HSV. Ad-UI1 showed selective cytotoxicity against androgen-independent PSA/PSMA-expressing prostate cancer cells in preclinical models of PCa [53].

In another approach, a triplet of prostate-specific enhancers was constructed to regulate adenovirus replication generating Ad[I/PPT-E1A] with E1A under the control of a complex chimeric promoter/enhancer sequence designated PPT [54, 55]. PPT is comprised of the T-cell receptor γ-alternate reading frame protein promoter (TARP) and the PSMA and PSA enhancers.

The chimeric sequence is shielded from interfering adenoviral promoter-sequences by the mouse H19 insulator. Ad[I/PPT-E1A] demonstrated high and prostate-specific replication both in the presence and absence of androgens with promising oncolytic effects in PCa cell lines. Moreover, LNCaP xenograft tumours in mice regressed after intratumoural administration of Ad[I/PPT-E1A].

3.4. Targeted replication of adenovirus through complementation deletions

Several modified versions of Onyx-015 have been designed to develop prostate-specific onco-lytic adenoviruses [15, 56]. For example, Ad5-CD/TKrep is armed with the cytosine deaminase (CD) and TK suicide genes [57]. In a phase I study, the intratumoural administration of Ad5-CD/TKrep was evaluated in locally recurrent prostate cancer in combination with the prodrugs 5-fluorocytosine (5-FC) and ganciclovir [20]. Ad5-CD/TKrep reduced PSA levels with a good safety profile; 44% of patients showed more than 25% decreases in PSA and 19% showed more than 50% decreases in PSA. Tumour cell killing at the administration sites was demonstrated by biopsies 2 weeks later. Interestingly, two patients were cancer free at 1 year follow-up.

Later, a second-generation of Ad5-CD/TKrep was developed; Ad5-yCD/mutTKSR39rep-ADP expressing the adenovirus death protein (ADP) and an improved yeast CD/TK chimeric suicide construct [58]. Ad5-yCD/mutTKSR39rep-ADP showed higher cancer cell killing activity in pre-clinical studies compared to the parental virus. Moreover, in a phase II trial, promising synergis-tic anticancer activity was seen in combination with radiation therapy [21]. Another version of this mutant is (Ad5-yCD/mutTKSR39rep-hNIS), which in addition to the chimeric suicide gene expresses the human sodium iodide symporter (hNIS), which serves as a reporter gene to enable localisation through noninvasive single-photon emission computed tomography (SPECT/CT) [59]. The most recent version of these mutants is Ad5-yCD/mutTKSR39rep-hIL12, which instead of hNIS expresses the human interleukin 12 (IL-12) [60]. IL-12 is a proinflammatory cytokine released by antigen-presenting cells to activate the innate and adaptive immune responses. IL-12 has reported antitumour activity by overcoming the immune suppressive nature of the tumour microenvironment and inhibiting angiogenesis. Local administration of Ad5-yCD/mutTKSR-39rep-hIL12 may evade systemic toxicity of IL-12 while maintaining its therapeutic activity locally. Systemic administration of Ad5/3Δ24hCG, targeting the Ad3 receptor expresses the β-chain of human chorionic gonadotropin (hCGβ), was reported to have anticancer activity in mice with castration-resistant lung metastasis of PCa, resulting in significant survival advantages [43].

4. Challenges using oncolytic adenoviruses for prostate cancer

The promising results from clinical trials with oncolytic adenoviral mutants are, in the majority of cases, derived from localised PCa and intratumoural administration [18, 20, 21]. However, the poor survival outcomes for late-stage PCa patients are due to metastatic lesions in skel-eton and lymph nodes. While the oncolytic mutants readily spread within the tumour tissue after local administration, metastatic lesions need to be targeted through systemic delivery, which is currently not feasible due to the high-affinity binding to erythrocytes, other factors present in the blood, and through elimination of virus from the circulation by the liver [8, 61].

4.1. Preexisting antibodies

A major hurdle in achieving efficient tumour uptake after systemic delivery of oncolytic ade-noviruses is the preexisting immunity to virus since the majority of the population has previ-ously been infected with adenovirus. One strategy to overcome preexisitng immunity is to encapsulate the virus in liposomes. It was demonstrated that despite the presence of adenovi-rus antibodies, liposome-coated virus infected tumour cells in preclinical *in vivo* models [62]. Another strategy, which has also been explored in noncancer research, is the administration of anti-CD20 antibodies to inhibit T cells and deplete B cells from the host. This strategy resulted in enhanced replication of adenoviruses regardless of preexisting adenoviral immunity [63]. A more sophisticated approach is the "Trojan Horse", in which the virus is delivered within a host cell that targets tumours. A similar approach is incorporation of the E1A gene into cyto-toxic T lymphocytes (CTL) with expression controlled by the cell activation-dependent CD40 ligand promoter [64]. After transduction of CTLs with E1-deficient adenoviral vectors and activation by CD40, E1A was expressed and infectious virus was produced. Viral replication was tightly associated with CTL activation by its specific tumour-associated antigen, resulting in targeted delivery of oncolytic virus to the tumour [64].

4.2. Binding to erythrocytes

Human erythrocytes express CAR and complement receptor-1 (CR1) that bind to adenovirus with high affinity [65]. The binding significantly decreases the levels of free circulating virus, in turn attenuating viral infection of tumour target tissue. Therefore, erythrocyte binding is a great challenge for systemic administration of oncolytic adenoviruses. To overcome these obstacles, it might be possible to shield the virus with a layer of hydrophilic polyethylene glycol, modifica-tions of the capsid proteins, or as described above with liposome encapsulation [62, 66].

4.3. Uptake by nontargeted healthy tissue

Most adenoviruses are eliminated from the circulation by Kupffer cells through nonreceptor-mediated uptake [67, 68]. For Ad5, up to 90% is taken up by hepatocytes and Kupffer cells in the liver within minutes of intravenous delivery in humans, drastically preventing sufficient amount of virus to reach the targeted tumours [68]. To increase the amount of circulating virus, several strategies have been investigated. One preclinical study explored preadmin-istration of warfarin, which depleted Kupffer cells and prevented hepatocyte binding and consequently improved the anticancer activity of an intravenously administered oncolytic adenovirus [69]. Although warfarin administration may not be feasible in patients, the study demonstrated that circulating levels of Ad5 mutants could be increased by blocking liver uptake. The major key factors associated with liver sequestration of oncolytic Ad5 mutants are the blood coagulation factors IX (FIX) and X (FX) that bind to the capsid proteins and mediate erythrocyte and hepatocyte binding [70]. To avoid these interactions, various chi-meric capsid mutants have been generated with altered hexon and/or fibre proteins includ-ing the Ad3/Ad11 mutant ColoAd1 (enadenotucirev; PsiOxus) that is currently in phase I–II trials with reported promising outcomes in several solid cancers after systemic delivery [71]. Another mutant Ad5/48 with hexon proteins from Ad48, which have low affinity to FX, dem-onstrated decreased liver uptake in preclinical models [72].

4.4. Endogenous cytokines

Systemic virus administration stimulates the release of a range of cytokines such as interferons (IFN types 1, 2, and 3) [73]. Their major roles are to induce apoptosis of virus-infected cells and promote resistance to infection in noninfected cells. Moreover, IFNs stimulate the adaptive immune system, mainly the dendritic cells, to initiate long-term immunity. One strategy to overcome the IFN-response is to pretreat the patients with histone deacetylase inhibitors (HDACi) that induce epigenetic changes preventing antiviral cytokine activity at the tumour sites and significantly enhancing systemic efficacy of oncolytic mutants [74]. Delivery of the virus within mesenchymal stem cells derived from the patient may also aid in avoiding the IFN responses since mesenchymal stem cells suppress activated T cells [75].

5. Future directions

The efficacy of numerous oncolytic viruses in cancer management has been established, although only two mutants have been granted market approval to date [15, 17]. Major clinical drawbacks associated with oncolytic adenoviruses are the significant losses of virus after systemic administration resulting in low doses reaching the tumour lesions. In addition, the complexity of designing potent and selective oncolytic viruses without toxicity to normal cells but potent cancer killing activity requires further optimisations. Ongoing work is focused on all aspects of delivering optimised mutants to metastatic lesions. One novel approach is to employ less common serotypes, including Ad3, Ad11, and Ad48, that are more resistant to elimination after intravenous administration. Natural infection with these serotypes is less frequent and preexisting immunity is rare. In addition, the utilisation of other uptake receptors than those of Ad5, CAR, and $\alpha v \beta 3$- and $\alpha v \beta 5$-integrins is an advantage both for improved cancer-cell uptake and decreased erythrocyte and blood-factor binding. A similar approach is the use of chimeric adenoviral mutants including replication-selective alterations of, for example, the Ad5 genome and exchange of capsid proteins from other serotypes such as Ad3 and Ad11. A method for generating cancer cell–selective optimised novel chimeric mutants is "directed evolution" [75]. This concept involves pooling of several serotypes of adenovirus followed by numerous passaging of virus on the cancer cell type of interest, which promotes recombination between serotypes. This process represents an accelerated simulation of the natural selection of viruses, and the most potent mutant can be selected from the resultant viral pools for further study. The methodology can be applied to most epithelial cancer cell lines. To date, a potent oncolytic adenovirus has been generated using this approach, ColoAd1 (enadenotucirev; PsiOxus), which entered phase I–II trials with reported promising outcomes in several solid cancers after systemic delivery [71]. Potency and selectivity on colon cancer cells were significantly higher compared to Onyx-015 [76]. ColoAd1 was selected on colon cancer cell lines and was not evaluated in PCa patients; however, a similar approach using prostate cancer cell lines may lead to the generation of prostate-selective chimeric adenoviruses suitable for systemic administration.

A major advantage of using adenoviruses as anticancer therapeutics is the safety with only self-limiting flu-like side effects [77]. While administration of current oncolytic adenoviral mutants as single agents has not resulted in significant increases in survival, in combination with cytotoxic drugs and immune factors, efficacy was greatly improved [7, 48]. One strategy to overcome the high level of resistance to anticancer immune responses is to include trans-genes into the viral genome, such as GM-CSF and IL-12, to further improve the anticancer activity by boosting antitumour immunity [8, 78]. Arming oncolytic viruses with immune stimulatory factors show promise since intralesional administration of virus might induce a synergistic action between viral oncolysis and antitumour immune responses. This concept is particularly significant for prostate cancer management, as prostate cancer usually does not respond to management with immunotherapeutic agents such as check point inhibitors, due to the immunosuppressive character of this cancer [79]. In addition, the immune responses resulting from cancer cell lysis and death are anticipated to target metastatic tumours even after clearance of the oncolytic virus from the body.

Other issues are the variable susceptibility of tumours to oncolytic adenoviral mutants, likely caused by the specific gene alterations in each tumour type [80]. It may be possible to char-acterise each patient tumour and select from a panel of oncolytic adenoviruses specifically targeting the identified mutations. A more practical approach to enhance oncolytic efficacy is through combining the mutants with other treatment modalities including cytotoxic drugs and small molecule–targeted therapies [80, 81]. A recent example is the combination of the H101 mutant with a small interfering RNA targeting Bcl2 (siBcl2) [80]. In preclinical studies, the combination resulted in significantly increased tumour cell cytotoxicity and apoptosis compared to either agent alone. *In vivo* tumour xenograft studies demonstrated that combin-ing H101 with siBcl2 significantly reduced tumour growth and prolonged survival.

6. Conclusions

For patients with early-stage prostate cancer, the current treatment modalities are efficient, with 5-year progression-free survival rates of more than 90%. On the other hand, for patients with advanced PCa (stages III and IV), there is currently no effective therapy. Although the latest therapeutic developments for late-stage metastatic PCa have provided a variety of man-agement options that offer significant clinical benefits for patients, the disease still has almost 100% mortality rate at this stage. The median survival after development of hormone resis-tance is 14 months. Current treatment options have modest effects on survival, extending life by around 2.5–5 months, and are associated with increased treatment costs [82]. Therefore, the need for novel therapies is pressing. Oncolytic viruses have proven potential for the future management of PCa. Several factors make adenoviruses valuable anticancer agents, such as the biology of the viruses is well understood, the viral genome is small and easy to manip-ulate, and the viruses can induce direct cell death, synergise with apoptosis-inducing che-motherapeutic drugs and stimulate the immune system to develop cancer-specific immune responses. The anticancer mechanisms of adenoviruses are unique without the development of cross-resistance to current therapeutics and have only mild side effects.

Adenoviruses are the most attractive and promising oncolytic virus species that have yet been developed for treatment of different types of solid cancers including PCa. Reports from phase I–II clinical trials, including PCa patients, demonstrate that these viruses have excellent safety profiles that have been reproduced in thousands of patients. The reported efficacy is promising because of the synergistic interactions between oncolytic adenoviruses and chemotherapy/radiotherapy. Phase III clinical trials are ongoing to assess the efficacy of oncolytic mutants in locally recurrent and high-risk local prostate cancers [21]. If the results of these trials confirm the efficacy and safety, the first oncolytic virus therapy for PCa patients may become a reality in the future. Additionally, arming the viruses with cytotoxic transgenes and immune stimulatory factors represents a promising approach to enhance efficacy in both localised and metastatic PCa. A recent advancement in the development of optimised oncolytic viruses is the generation of chimeric viruses by utilising serotypes that are more resistant in the circulation. An effective but labour-intense approach is to generate chimeric oncolytic adenovirus with enhanced potency, circulating half-life and selectivity to specific cancer types by directed evolution [76]. The major drawback of oncolytic adenoviruses is the disappointing anticancer activity against distant metastatic tumours after systemic administration, and by employing novel chimeric serotypes, it may be possible to develop superior mutants with properties suitable for intravenous delivery. The adenoviral mutants Ad5/3Δ24hCG demonstrated promising anticancer activity in preclinical metastatic hormone-resistant PCa models, which prolonged survival *in vivo* [43]. If the same results are reproduced in patients, a great impact on the management of metastatic PCa can be anticipated. We predict that in the near future oncolytic adenoviruses will be a treatment choice for this indication and will add to the novel therapies that aim to cure late-stage castration-resistant prostate cancer.

Author details

Ahmed A. Ali and Gunnel Halldén*

*Address all correspondence to: g.hallden@qmul.ac.uk

Centre for Molecular Oncology, Barts Cancer Institute, Queen Mary University of London, London, UK

References

[1] American Cancer Society. Information and Resources about for Cancer: Breast, Colon, Lung, Prostate, Skin. 2017. Available from: https://www.cancer.org/cancer/prostate-cancer/detection-diagnosis-staging/survival-rates.html

[2] Marberger M, Barentsz J, Emberton M, Hugosson J, Loeb S, Klotz L, et al. Novel approaches to improve prostate cancer diagnosis and management in early-stage disease. BJU International. 2012;**109**(Suppl 2):1-7

[3] Clegg NJ, Wongvipat J, Joseph J, Tran C, Ouk S, Dilhas A, et al. ARN-509: A novel antiandrogen for prostate cancer treatment. Cancer Research. 2012;**72**(6):1494-1503

[4]   Harland S, Staffurth J, Molina A, Hao Y, Gagnon DD, Sternberg CN, et al. Effect of abi-raterone acetate treatment on the quality of life of patients with metastatic castration-resistant prostate cancer after failure of docetaxel chemotherapy. European Journal of Cancer. 2013;**49**(17):3648-3657

[5]   Delwar Z, Zhang K, Rennie PS, Jia W. Oncolytic virotherapy for urological cancers. Nature Reviews. Urology. 2016;**13**(6):334-352

[6]   Nguyen A, Ho L, Wan Y. Chemotherapy and oncolytic virotherapy: Advanced tactics in the war against cancer. Frontiers in Oncology. 2014;**4**(145):1-10

[7]   Yu DC, Chen Y, Dilley J, Li Y, Embry M, Zhang H, et al. Antitumor synergy of CV787, a prostate cancer-specific adenovirus, and paclitaxel and docetaxel. Cancer Research. 2001;**61**(2):517-525

[8]   Sweeney K, Halldén G. Oncolytic adenovirus-mediated therapy for prostate cancer. Oncolytic Virotherapy. 2016;**5**:45-57

[9]   Parato KA, Senger D, Forsyth PA, Bell JC. Recent progress in the battle between oncolytic viruses and tumours. Nature Reviews. Cancer. 2005;**5**(12):965-976

[10] Fukuhara H, Ino Y, Todo T. Oncolytic virus therapy: A new era of cancer treatment at dawn. Cancer Science. 2016;**107**(10):1373-1379

[11] Huebner RJ, Rowe WP, Schatten WE, Smith RR, Thomas LB. Studies on the use of viruses in the treatment of carcinoma of the cervix. Cancer. 1956;**9**(6):1211-1218

[12] Kelly E, Russell SJ. History of oncolytic viruses: Genesis to genetic engineering. Molecular Therapy. 2007;**15**(4):651-659

[13] Platanias LC. Mechanisms of type-I- and type-II-interferon-mediated signalling. Nature Reviews. Immunology. 2005;**5**(5):375-386

[14] Martuza RL, Malick A, Markert JM, Ruffner KL, Coen DM. Experimental therapy of human glioma by means of a genetically engineered virus mutant. Science. 1991;**252**(5007):854-856

[15] Heise C, Sampson-Johannes A, Williams A, McCormick F, Von Hoff DD, Kirn DH. ONYX-015, an E1B gene-attenuated adenovirus, causes tumor-specific cytolysis and antitumoral efficacy that can be augmented by standard chemotherapeutic agents. Nature Medicine. 1997;**3**(6):639-645

[16] Garber K. China approves world's first oncolytic virus therapy for cancer treatment. Journal of the National Cancer Institute. 2006;**98**:298-300

[17] Coffin R. Interview with Robert coffin, inventor of T-VEC: The first oncolytic immuno-therapy approved for the treatment of cancer. Immunotherapy. 2016;**8**(2):103-106

[18] TL DW, van der Poel H, Li S, Mikhak B, Drew R, Goemann M, et al. A phase I trial of CV706, a replication-competent, PSA selective oncolytic adenovirus, for the treat-ment of locally recurrent prostate cancer following radiation therapy. Cancer Research. 2001;**61**(20):7464-7472

[19] Small EJ, Carducci MA, Burke JM, Rodriguez R, Fong L, van Ummersen L, et al. A phase I trial of intravenous CG7870, a replication-selective, prostate-specific antigen-targeted oncolytic adenovirus, for the treatment of hormone-refractory, metastatic prostate cancer. Molecular Therapy. 2006;14(1):107-117

[20] Freytag SO, Khil M, Stricker H, Peabody J, Menon M, DePeralta-Venturina M, et al. Phase I study of replication-competent adenovirus-mediated double suicide gene therapy for the treatment of locally recurrent prostate cancer. Cancer Research. 2002;62(17):4968-4976

[21] Freytag SO, Stricker H, Lu M, Elshaikh M, Aref I, Pradhan D, et al. Prospective randomized phase 2 trial of intensity modulated radiation therapy with or without oncolytic adenovirus-mediated cytotoxic gene therapy in intermediate-risk prostate cancer. International Journal of Radiation Oncology, Biology, Physics. 2014;89(2):268-276

[22] Vidal L, Pandha HS, Yap TA, White CL, Twigger K, Vile RG, et al. A phase I study of intravenous oncolytic reovirus type 3 dearing in patients with advanced cancer. Clinical Cancer Research. 2008;14(21):7127-7137

[23] Comins C, Spicer J, Protheroe A, Roulstone V, Twigger K, White CM, et al. REO-10: A phase I study of intravenous reovirus and docetaxel in patients with advanced cancer. Clinical Cancer Research. 2010;16(22):5564-5572

[24] Rowe WP, Huebner RJ, Gilmore LK, Parrott RH, Ward TG. Isolation of a cytopathogenic agent from human adenoids undergoing spontaneous degeneration in tissue culture. Proceedings of the Society for Experimental Biology and Medicine. 1953;84(3):570-573

[25] Ghebremedhin B. Human adenovirus: Viral pathogen with increasing importance. European Journal of Microbiology and Immunology. 2014;4(1):26-33

[26] Larson C, Oronsky B, Scicinski J, Fanger GR, Stirn M, Oronsky A, et al. Going viral: A review of replication-selective oncolytic adenoviruses. Oncotarget. 2015;6(24):19976-19989

[27] Goldufsky J, Sivendran S, Harcharik S, Pan M, Bernardo S, Stern RH, et al. Oncolytic virus therapy for cancer. Oncolytic Virotherapy. 2013;2:31-46

[28] Fields BN, Knipe DM, Howley PM. Fields Virology. Adenoviruses. Chapter 67. Philadelphia: Wolters Kluwer Health/Lippincott Williams & Wilkins; 2007. pp. 2265-2300

[29] Saha B, Wong CM, Parks RJ. The adenovirus genome contributes to the structural stability of the Virion. Virus. 2014;6(9):3563-3583

[30] Davison AJ, Benko M, Harrach B. Genetic content and evolution of adenoviruses. The Journal of General Virology. 2003;84(Pt 11):2895-2908

[31] Fields BN, Knipe DM, Howley PM. Fields Virology. Adenoviruses. Chapter 68. Philadelphia: Wolters Kluwer Health/Lippincott Williams & Wilkins; 2007. pp. 2301-2326

[32] Waye MMY, Sing CW. Anti-viral drugs for human adenoviruses. Pharmaceuticals (Basel). 2010;3(10):3343-3354

[33] Zielinski T, Jordan E. Remote results of clinical observation of the oncolytic action of adenoviruses on cervix cancer. Nowotwory. 1969;19(3):217-221

[34] Krasnykh V, Dmitriev I, Mikheeva G, Miller CR, Belousova N, Curiel DT. Characterization of an adenovirus vector containing a heterologous peptide epitope in the HI loop of the fiber knob. Journal of Virology. 1998;**72**(3):1844-1852

[35] Gamble LJ, Borovjagin AV, Matthews QL. Role of RGD-containing ligands in targeting cellular integrins: Applications for ovarian cancer virotherapy. Experimental and Therapeutic Medicine. 2010;**1**(2):233-240

[36] Takayama K, Reynolds PN, Short JJ, Kawakami Y, Adachi Y, Glasgow JN, et al. A mosaic adenovirus possessing serotype Ad5 and serotype Ad3 knobs exhibits expanded tropism. Virology. 2003;**309**(2):282-293

[37] Ulasov IV, Rivera AA, Han Y, Curiel DT, Zhu ZB, Lesniak MS. Targeting adenovirus to CD80 and CD86 receptors increases gene transfer efficiency to malignant glioma cells. Journal of Neurosurgery. 2007;**107**(3):617-627

[38] Stevenson SC, Rollence M, Marshall-Neff J, McClelland A. Selective targeting of human cells by a chimeric adenovirus vector containing a modified fiber protein. Journal of Virology. 1997;**71**(6):4782-4790

[39] Kwon OJ, Kang E, Choi JW, Kim SW, Yun CO. Therapeutic targeting of chitosan-PEG-folate-complexed oncolytic adenovirus for active and systemic cancer gene therapy. Journal of Controlled Release. 2013 Aug 10;**169**(3):257-265

[40] Rivlin N, Brosh R, Oren M, Rotter V. Mutations in the p53 tumor suppressor gene: Important milestones at the various steps of tumorigenesis. Genes & Cancer. 2011;**2**(4): 466-474

[41] O'Shea CC, Johnson L, Bagus B, Choi S, Nicholas C, Shen A, et al. Late viral RNA export, rather than p53 inactivation, determines ONYX-015 tumor selectivity. Cancer Cell. 2004;**6**(6):611-623

[42] Page JG, Tian B, Schweikart K, Tomaszewski J, Harris R, Broadt T, et al. Identifying the safety profile of a novel infectivity-enhanced conditionally replicative adenovirus, Ad5-delta24-RGD, in anticipation of a phase I trial for recurrent ovarian cancer. American Journal of Obstetrics and Gynecology. 2007;**196**(4):389.e1-389.e9 discussion .e9-10

[43] Rajecki M, Kanerva A, Stenman UH, Tenhunen M, Kangasniemi L, Sarkioja M, et al. Treatment of prostate cancer with Ad5/3Delta24hCG allows non-invasive detection of the magnitude and persistence of virus replication in vivo. Molecular Cancer Therapeutics. 2007;**6**(2):742-751

[44] Rodriguez R, Schuur ER, Lim HY, Henderson GA, Simons JW, Henderson DR. Prostate attenuated replication competent adenovirus (ARCA) CN706: A selective cytotoxic for prostate-specific antigen-positive prostate cancer cells. Cancer Research. 1997;**57**(13): 2559-2563

[45] Li X, Zhang YP, Kim HS, Bae KH, Stantz KM, Lee SJ, et al. Gene therapy for prostate cancer by controlling adenovirus E1a and E4 gene expression with PSES enhancer. Cancer Research. 2005;**65**(5):1941-1951

[46] Wu L, Matherly J, Smallwood A, Adams JY, Billick E, Belldegrun A, et al. Chimeric PSA enhancers exhibit augmented activity in prostate cancer gene therapy vectors. Gene Therapy. 2001;**8**(18):1416-1426

[47] Yu DC, Chen Y, Seng M, Dilley J, Henderson DR. The addition of adenovirus type 5 region E3 enables calydon virus 787 to eliminate distant prostate tumor xenografts. Cancer Research. 1999;**59**(17):4200-4203

[48] Dilley J, Reddy S, Ko D, Nguyen N, Rojas G, Working P, et al. Oncolytic adenovirus CG7870 in combination with radiation demonstrates synergistic enhancements of anti-tumor efficacy without loss of specificity. Cancer Gene Therapy. 2005;**12**(8):715-722

[49] Wilding G, Carducci M, Yu DC, Burke J, Borellini F, Aimi J, et al. A phase 1/11 trial of IV CG7870, a replication-selective, PSA-targeted oncolytic adenovirus (OAV), for the treatment of hormone-refractory, metastatic prostate cancer. Journal of Clinical Oncology. 2004;**22**(14_suppl):3036

[50] Ghosh A, Heston WD. Tumor target prostate specific membrane antigen (PSMA) and its regulation in prostate cancer. Journal of Cellular Biochemistry. 2004;**91**(3):528-539

[51] Watt F, Martorana A, Brookes DE, Ho T, Kingsley E, O'Keefe DS, et al. A tissue-specific enhancer of the prostate-specific membrane antigen gene, FOLH1. Genomics. 2001;**73**(3):243-254

[52] Lee SJ, Zhang Y, Lee SD, Jung C, Li X, Kim HS, et al. Targeting prostate cancer with conditionally replicative adenovirus using PSMA enhancer. Molecular Therapy. 2004;**10**(6):1051-1058

[53] Ahn M, Lee SJ, Li X, Jiménez J, Zhang YP, Bae KH, et al. Enhanced combined tumor-specific oncolysis and suicide gene therapy for prostate cancer using M6 promoter. Cancer Gene Therapy. 2009;**16**(1):73-82

[54] Cheng WS, Dzojic H, Nilsson B, Totterman TH, Essand M. An oncolytic conditionally replicating adenovirus for hormone-dependent and hormone-independent prostate cancer. Cancer Gene Therapy. 2006;**13**(1):13-20

[55] Cheng WS, Kraaij R, Nilsson B, van der Weel L, de Ridder CM, Totterman TH, et al. A novel TARP-promoter-based adenovirus against hormone-dependent and hormone-refractory prostate cancer. Molecular Therapy. 2004;**10**(2):355-364

[56] Bischoff JR, Kirn DH, Williams A, Heise C, Horn S, Muna M, et al. An adenovirus mutant that replicates selectively in p53-deficient human tumor cells. Science. 1996;**274**(5286):373-376

[57] Freytag SO, Rogulski KR, Paielli DL, Gilbert JD, Kim JH. A novel three-pronged approach to kill cancer cells selectively: Concomitant viral, double suicide gene, and radiotherapy. Human Gene Therapy. 1998;**9**(9):1323-1333

[58] Barton KN, Paielli D, Zhang Y, Koul S, Brown SL, Lu M, et al. Second-generation replication-competent oncolytic adenovirus armed with improved suicide genes and ADP gene demonstrates greater efficacy without increased toxicity. Molecular Therapy. 2006;**13**(2):347-356

[59] Barton KN, Stricker H, Elshaikh MA, Pegg J, Cheng J, Zhang Y, et al. Feasibility of adenovirus-mediated hNIS gene transfer and 131I radioiodine therapy as a definitive treatment for localized prostate cancer. Molecular Therapy. 2011;**19**(7):1353-1359

[60] Freytag SO, Zhang Y, Siddiqui F. Preclinical toxicology of oncolytic adenovirus-mediated cytotoxic and interleukin-12 gene therapy for prostate cancer. Molecular Therapy — Oncolytics. 2015;**2**:15006. DOI: 10.1038/mto.2015.6

[61] Ferguson MS, Lemoine NR, Wang Y. Systemic delivery of oncolytic viruses: Hopes and hurdles. Advances in Virology. 2012. DOI: 10.1155/2012/805629

[62] Yotnda P, Davis AR, Hicks MJ, Templeton NS, Brenner MK. Liposomal enhancement of the antitumor activity of conditionally replication-competent adenoviral plasmids. Molecular Therapy. 2004;**9**(4):489-495

[63] Fontanellas A, Hervas-Stubbs S, Mauleon I, Dubrot J, Mancheno U, Collantes M, et al. Intensive pharmacological immunosuppression allows for repetitive liver gene transfer with recombinant adenovirus in nonhuman primates. Molecular Therapy. 2010;**18**(4):754-765

[64] Yotnda P, Savoldo B, Charlet-Berguerand N, Rooney C, Brenner M. Targeted delivery of adenoviral vectors by cytotoxic T cells. Blood. 2004;**104**(8):2272-2280

[65] Carlisle RC, Di Y, Cerny AM, Sonnen AF, Sim RB, Green NK, et al. Human erythrocytes bind and inactivate type 5 adenovirus by presenting Coxsackie virus-adenovirus receptor and complement receptor 1. Blood. 2009;**113**(9):1909-1918

[66] Tian J, Xu Z, Smith JS, Hofherr SE, Barry MA, Byrnes AP. Adenovirus activates complement by distinctly different mechanisms in vitro and in vivo: Indirect complement activation by virions in vivo. Journal of Virology. 2009;**83**(11):5648-5658

[67] Alemany R, Suzuki K, Curiel DT. Blood clearance rates of adenovirus type 5 in mice. The Journal of General Virology. 2000;**81**(Pt 11):2605-2609

[68] Khare R, May SM, Vetrini F, Weaver EA, Palmer D, Rosewell A, et al. Generation of a Kupffer cell-evading adenovirus for systemic and liver-directed gene transfer. Molecular Therapy. 2011;**19**(7):1254-1262

[69] Shashkova EV, Doronin K, Senac JS, Barry MA. Macrophage depletion combined with anticoagulant therapy increases therapeutic window of systemic treatment with oncolytic adenovirus. Cancer Research. 2008;**68**(14):5896-5904

[70] Jonsson MI, Lenman AE, Frängsmyr L, Nyberg C, Abdullahi M, Arnberg N. Coagulation factors IX and X enhance binding and infection of adenovirus types 5 and 31 in human epithelial cells. Journal of Virology. 2009;**83**(8):3816-3825

[71] Garcia-Carbonero R, Salazar R, Duran I, Osman-Garcia I, Paz-Ares L, Bozada JM, et al. Phase 1 study of intravenous administration of the chimeric adenovirus enadenotucirev in patients undergoing primary tumor resection. Journal of Immunotherpay of Cancer. 2017;**5**(71). DOI: 10.1186/s40425-017-0277-7

[72] Zhang Z, Krimmel J, Hu Z, Seth P. Systemic delivery of a novel liver-detargeted onco-lytic adenovirus causes reduced liver toxicity but maintains the antitumor response in a breast cancer bone metastasis model. Human Gene Therapy. 2011;**22**(9):1137-1142

[73] Randall RE, Goodbourn S. Interferons and viruses: An interplay between induction, sig-nalling, antiviral responses and virus countermeasures. The Journal of General Virology. 2008;**89**(Pt 1):1-47

[74] Nguyen TL, Abdelbary H, Arguello M, Breitbach C, Leveille S, Diallo JS, et al. Chemical targeting of the innate antiviral response by histone deacetylase inhibitors renders refractory cancers sensitive to viral oncolysis. Proceedings of the National Academy of Sciences of the United States of America. 2008;**105**(39):14981-14986

[75] Ahmed AU, Rolle CE, Tyler MA, Han Y, Sengupta S, Wainwright DA, et al. Bone marrow mesenchymal stem cells loaded with an oncolytic adenovirus suppress the anti-adenovi-ral immune response in the cotton rat model. Molecular Therapy. 2010;**18**(10):1846-1856

[76] Kuhn I, Harden P, Bauzon M, Chartier C, Nye J, Thorne S, et al. Directed evolution gener-ates a novel oncolytic virus for the treatment of colon cancer. PLoS One. 2008;**3**(6):e2409

[77] Buijs PR, Verhagen JH, van Eijck CH, van den Hoogen BG. Oncolytic viruses: From bench to bedside with a focus on safety. Human Vaccines & Immunotherapeutics. 2015;**11**(7): 1573-1584

[78] Uusi-Kerttula H, Hulin-Curtis S, Davies J, Parker AL. Oncolytic adenovirus: Strategies and insights for vector design and immuno-oncolytic applications. Virus. 2015;**7**(11): 6009-6042

[79] Kwon ED, Drake CG, Scher HI, Fizazi K, Bossi A, van den Eertwegh AJ, et al. Ipilimumab versus placebo after radiotherapy in patients with metastatic castration-resistant pros-tate cancer that had progressed after docetaxel chemotherapy (CA184-043): A multicen-tre, randomised, double-blind, phase 3 trial. The Lancet Oncology. 2014;**15**(7):700-712

[80] Zhang H, Wang H, Zhang J, Qian G, Niu B, Fan X, et al. Enhanced therapeutic effi-cacy by simultaneously targeting two genetic defects in Tumors. Molecular Therapy. 2008;**17**(1):57-64

[81] Simpson GR, Relph K, Harrington K, Melcher A, Pandha H. Cancer immunotherapy via combining oncolytic virotherapy with chemotherapy: Recent advances. Oncolytic Virotherapy. 2016;**5**:1-13

[82] Kirby M, Hirst C, Crawford ED. Characterising the castration-resistant prostate cancer population: A systematic review. International Journal of Clinical Practice. 2011;**65**(11): 1180-1192